A PHYSIOLOGICAL
APPROACH TO
CLINICAL
NEUROLOGY

A
Physiological Approach

James W. Lance
M.D., M.R.C.P., F.R.A.C.P

By the same author
The Mechanism and Management of Headache

to Clinical Neurology

Chairman, Division of Neurology,
Prince Henry and Prince of Wales
Hospitals; Associate Professor of
Medicine, University of New South
Wales, Sydney, Australia

London: Butterworths

ENGLAND: BUTTERWORTH & CO. (PUBLISHERS) LTD.
                    LONDON: 88 Kingsway, W.C.2
AUSTRALIA: BUTTERWORTH & CO. (AUSTRALIA) LTD.
                    SYDNEY: 20 Loftus Street
                    MELBOURNE: 343 Little Collins Street
                    BRISBANE: 240 Queen Street
CANADA: BUTTERWORTH & CO. (CANADA) LTD.
                    TORONTO: 14 Curity Avenue, 374
NEW ZEALAND: BUTTERWORTH & CO. (NEW ZEALAND) LTD.
                    WELLINGTON: 49/51 Ballance Street
                    AUCKLAND: 35 High Street
SOUTH AFRICA: BUTTERWORTH & CO. (SOUTH AFRICA) LTD.
                    DURBAN: 33/35 Beach Grove

Suggested U.D.C. No. 612·8:616·8

ISBN 0 407 35850 1

Printed in Great Britain by
R. J. Acford Ltd., Industrial Estate, Chichester, Sussex

To Professor P. O. Bishop
who must assume some responsibility for my becoming
a neurologist

Contents

Preface

As a clinical neurologist and amateur physiologist, I have always
sought to bridge the gap between the research laboratory and the
hospital ward in teaching undergraduate and postgraduate students.
A knowledge of neuroanatomy and neuropathology is generally
accepted as a basis for the understanding of clinical neurology,
while neurophysiology has become isolated in the student's mind by
its technology, its emphasis on animal experimentation, and its
apparent lack of relevance to clinical problems. The account given
here attempts to overcome this unhappy state by explaining the
mechanism of various neurological symptoms and signs in terms of
disordered physiology wherever this is possible.

To present a simple version of complex and often controversial
mechanisms and then to illustrate the concept by line diagrams is to
invite criticism, but this has been done deliberately since the value of
an interpretation lies in its clarity as well as its validity. The validity
of the text will certainly change with the acquisition of new experimental evidence and re-examination of the old. Thus, no statement
in the following pages can be regarded as immutable. The coverage
is patchy, reflecting the interests and bias of the author, since there is
no intention to compete with comprehensive textbooks of neurophysiology or clinical neurology.

The first two chapters are designed as an introduction to the
clinical analysis of sensory and motor disorders. In the later chapters,
appraisal of current neurophysiological thought is applied to common
neurological syndromes. The author hopes that the presentation will
be clear enough to hold the interest of the clinical reader, without
being so artless as to offend the professional physiologist. The book
is proffered to those who are proceeding into the clinical years of a

medical course, to those who are studying for senior qualifications in internal medicine or neurology, and to those who are merely curious about the cause of neurological phenomena which they observe daily in their patients. However brilliant the physiological advances made in the understanding of other species, they are profitless for man until applied to him.

JAMES W. LANCE

Acknowledgements

I am indebted to Professor P. O. Bishop and Dr. J. G. McLeod for their helpful criticism of the text which has reduced, if not eliminated, its inadequacies. The continuation of the research programme into tonic and phasic stretch reflexes in man has only been possible through the assistance of Dr. J. D. Gillies, Dr. P. de Gail, Dr. C. A. Tassinari, Dr. D. Burke and Mr. P. D. Neilson, and financial support from the National Health and Medical Research Council of Australia, the Adolph Basser Foundation, Sandoz (Australia) Ltd. and Ciba Co. Pty. Ltd.

The preparation of the text owes much to my secretary, Mrs. R. M. Kendall, who has cheerfully added this task to her normal duties. Miss J. B. Pate, librarian, has kindly obtained all references for me.

The line diagrams were drawn by Mrs. G. Lindley from my primitive sketches, and all photographs and figures were prepared by the Department of Medical Illustration, University of New South Wales.

I am grateful to the editors of *Brain*, *Journal of Neurology, Neurosurgery and Psychiatry* and the *Medical Journal of Australia* for permission to use material and figures from earlier publications. I wish to thank those authors whose illustrations I have used as models, where acknowledged in the legends.

1—Pain and other Sensations

The nervous system of a normal individual is constantly active in conveying information to the brain about the state of the body and of the world outside it. If all these neuronal messages were received in equal measure, consciousness would become a nightmare of confused and largely irrelevant stimuli, so that a selective response would become impossible. Fortunately, there are various physiological processes which speed the passage of pertinent stimuli and retard awareness of the background activity. We thus become oblivious to the touch of clothes, the pressure of a hard seat and the functioning of contented viscera. The processes involved in this selectivity of sensations are as follows.

(1) Adaptation of sensory end organs, which cease to respond after variable periods of stimulation.

(2) Presynaptic inhibition of adjacent nerve cells by collaterals from an active nerve cell, thus assuring priority for 'the stimulus of the moment'[4]. This process probably takes place at all levels of the nervous system, thus repeatedly 'refining' the impulses representing a particular sensation, or, in electronic jargon, ensuring 'a high signal-to-noise ratio'.

(3) Regulation of synaptic transmission in sensory nuclei by the motor cortex. Stimulation of the sensorimotor cortex of the cat may inhibit or excite nerve cells in the cuneate and gracile nuclei by means of collaterals from the pyramidal tract and, to a lesser extent, by an extrapyramidal system[7, 21]. This provides a mechanism for the voluntary suppression of sensory information or for involuntary suppression during movement.

(4) Alteration in the state of awareness at a cortical level in that a subject while fully conscious, may so concentrate his

PAIN AND OTHER SENSATIONS

attention on a particular sensation, thought or response as to
preclude perception of other sensations.

The perception of any sensation therefore depends not only on the
appropriate receptor organ in skin, muscle, joint or viscus, and the
integrity of the peripheral nerve and spinal cord pathways, but also
on complex connexions within the cerebral cortex which may be
influenced by the thoughts and emotions of the subject. Thus sensation is subjective and each individual has his own 'perceptual world'
which is unique to him and can be known to others solely by his
description of it. A certain stimulus may be registered by some as
pleasant, by others as unpleasant but tolerable, and by others as so
uncomfortable that they use the term 'pain' to describe it. Each
person may therefore be regarded as having a 'pain threshold', and
if the level of sensory stimulation exceeds this, pain is experienced.

When the normal functioning of the body is disturbed, sensory
impulses of unusual quantity, quality or pattern are received by
the brain, and the resulting 'sense data' are expressed by the subject as
'symptoms'.

Sensory symptoms
Symptoms bring the patient to the doctor. It is part of the art of
medicine to record the patient's symptoms accurately and to interpret
them in the light of the patient's intellectual and educational endow-
ment, his personality and his emotional state.

Symptoms may be negative in that the patient complains of
numbness or inability to feel touch, pain, temperature or position of
the limbs. Symptoms may also be positive, providing curious
abnormal sensory experiences.

Ischaemia or irritation of peripheral nerves or the central projection of touch pathways gives rise to the prickling sensation described
as 'pins and needles' or the arm or leg 'going to sleep'. Compression
of the lateral cutaneous nerve of the thigh in the inguinal ligament
produces a curious creeping feeling in the outer aspect of the lower
thigh which has been likened to the sensation of ants crawling under
the skin (formication).

A disturbance within the posterior root entry zone or posterior
columns of the spinal cord, or pressure upon them, may be responsible
for a girdle sensation around the trunk, described as a tight band;
or a feeling of pressure in the limbs as though they were being
wrapped by a bandage. Sudden flexion of the neck may induce an
electric shock sensation which shoots down the back when there is a
cervical lesion irritating the posterior columns. This phenomenon
(Lhermitte's sign) is found most commonly in cervical spondylosis

2

and multiple sclerosis. A lesion in the spinothalamic tracts or thalamus produces an unpleasant burning sensation or pain which spreads diffusely down the opposite side of the body.

Irritation of the sensory cortex evokes paraesthesiae, which may spread rapidly over the contralateral side as an epileptic phenomenon, or advance more slowly when caused by migrainous vasospasm. The sensory association areas in the parietal lobe may give rise to weird illusions of the body image so that parts of the body appear larger or smaller than normal.

Pain is the most consistently unpleasant symptom which the nervous system can provide and may signal a disorder in any part of the body through irritation or distortion of sensory endorgans, or may arise from disease of the sensory pathways at any level from endorgan to cortex.

Pain is often associated with an emotional change so that it may be hard to determine which is primary and which secondary. In spite of all the complexities of the individual reaction to pain, it is usually possible to analyse the description of the pain so as to determine its site of origin and often its cause.

THE PERCEPTION OF DIFFERENT KINDS OF SENSATION: SEGREGATION OR INTEGRATION OF NEURAL PATHWAYS?

There is still controversy between those who believe that there are specific endorgans and nerve fibres for each modality of sensation, and those who believe that it is the pattern of impulses in any nerve which determines the type of sensation. The encapsulated endorgans which may serve a specialized function (touch, pressure, heat, cold) are concentrated in areas of the body which are particularly sensitive—the tips of the fingers, the lips, the areola of the breast and the genitalia. It is probable that all these endorgans may give rise to the sensation of pain if the stimulus is excessive. The free nerve endings which are found in profusion in all areas of skin are probably the chief pain receptors under normal circumstances, but it has been shown by Lele and Weddell[13] that even these may perceive sensations of touch, heat and cold as well.

Melzack and Wall[17] have put forward a hypothesis which attempts to unify the two conflicting concepts of sensibility. They point out that skin receptors are transducers which may respond to more than one type of environmental energy, and that the sequence of nerve impulses produced by the receptor is the function of a number of

3

physiological variables, such as the threshold to mechanical distortion, temperature change or chemical change, and the rate of adaptation to stimulation. The pattern of impulses entering the spinal cord from the periphery may be filtered out by the properties of the terminal branches of axons, which in turn will depend on activity in adjacent axons. Certain central cells may respond specifically to a temporal sequence of afferent impulses, a sudden increase and decrease in the case of a light pressure stimulus, or a steady low rate of bombardment in the case of change in skin temperature. The temporal pattern alone may not be sufficient to inform the central nervous system of the nature of the stimulus. Spatial summation from a large number of active fibres may then be required, particularly for pain sensation. Further refinement of sensation becomes possible because of the connexion of afferent fibres with specific central cells whose axons travel rostrally in pathways which transmit preferentially particular kinds of information.

This generalization still permits us to speak of 'pain pathways' or 'pain fibres' for the sake of simplicity although it is recognized that the association of various modalities with different groups of nerve fibres and nerve tracts is a loose one.

SENSORY PATHWAYS IN THE CENTRAL NERVOUS SYSTEM

Large afferent fibres from muscle spindles and tendon organs (group Ia and group Ib respectively) synapse in the posterior horns of the spinal cord and the second order neurones pass upwards mainly in the spinocerebellar tracts. There is comparatively little direct projection to the cerebral cortex, suggesting that their function lies in the regulation of motor activity rather than the conscious perception of muscular contraction. The perception of position of the limbs depends upon joint receptors.

Touch, light pressure and joint movement evoke discharges in fibres of smaller size than group I muscle afferents, which are conducted rostrally by neurones travelling in the posterior columns, (*Figure 1.1*). The majority of nerve fibres ascending in the posterior columns to reach the gracile and cuneate nuclei are first order neurones[19]. The second order neurones arise in these posterior column nuclei and cross over to pass upwards as the medial lemniscus to the external component of the thalamic ventrobasal complex (nucleus ventralis posterolateralis, VPL). The comparable fibres from the main sensory nucleus of the trigeminal nerve cross to join the lemniscal system and end in the arcuate or medial component of the

4

ventrobasal thalamic nuclei (nucleus ventralis posteromedialis, VPM).

The posterior column-lemniscal system appears to be responsible for the perception of joint position and the finer forms of tactile sensibility in man, which are tested clinically by stereognosis, two-point discrimination and figure-writing on the skin. The cerebral potentials which are evoked in man by stimulation of peripheral nerves also travel in the posterior columns and disappear in patients who have lost joint position sense, but not in those who have lost only pinprick and temperature sensation[5].

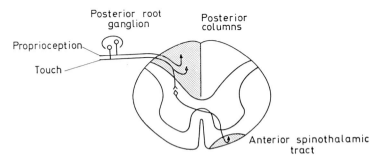

Figure 1.1 Spinal pathways for proprioception and touch (after Ranson, S. W. and Clark, S. L. (1959). 'Anatomy of the Nervous System'. Philadelphia and London; Saunders)

Fibres which are capable of serving the sensation of vibration are probably present in the lateral columns as well as the posterior columns, since vibration sense may be impaired with lesions of the lateral corticospinal tract and is sometimes preserved when joint position sense is lost[3]. Peripheral vibration suppresses cortical evoked potentials, probably by presynaptic inhibition at the spinal cord level (unpublished observations).

Some tactile sensations must be mediated by the spinothalamic system, because touch can still be perceived in man after damage to the posterior columns (*Figure 1.1*). This touch pathways of crossed second order neurones is known as the anterior spinothalamic tract, but its exact position in the anterolateral columns is unknown[19].

Temperature sensibility is thought to depend upon fibres of the delta group which synapse in the posterior horns of grey matter, the second order neurones crossing over within a few segments to ascend in the lateral spinothalamic tract in the same manner as those for pain sensation (*Figure 1.2*). The spinothalamic system is capable of considerable discrimination. Nathan and Rice[18] found that warm stimuli were localized less accurately than tactile stimuli, but that localization became more accurate as the intensity of stimulation increased to the point where the sensation of stinging or pricking became superimposed on that of warmth.

The perception of pain

Fibres from free nerve endings run in peripheral nerves to the posterior root and posterior horn of the spinal cord. There are two

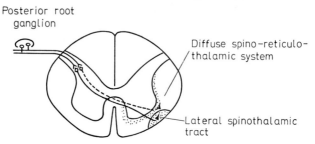

Posterior root ganglion

Diffuse spino-reticulo-thalamic system

Lateral spinothalamic tract

Figure 1.2. Spinal pathways for pain

groups of afferent fibres particularly associated with pain perception—unmyelinated fibres conducting slowly at 1–2 metres/second, and a group of myelinated fibres which conduct more rapidly at 10–20 metres/second. It is probable that the time interval in conduction between these two groups gives rise to the clinical phenomena of 'immediate' and 'delayed' pain[20].

Fibres involved in the transmission of pain sensation synapse in the posterior horn of grey matter in the spinal cord within a few segments of their entry into the cord and the second order neurones cross to the other side and then ascend in the lateral spinothalamic tract (*Figure 1.2*). It is now apparent that many pain fibres are scattered diffusely throughout the anterior and lateral white columns of the spinal cord, since it is necessary to destroy the greater part of this area before pain perception is abolished (*Figure 1.2*). These scattered 'extra-lemniscal fibres' relay in the reticular formation of the brain-stem, the intralaminar nuclei of the thalamus and the lateral reticular nucleus, and are distributed to both hemispheres by a diffuse thalamocortical projection[1], which is illustrated in *Figure 1.3*. The lateral spinothalamic tract is relayed by the nucleus ventralis posterolateralis (VPL) of the thalamus, and is projected to the sensory cortex in the post-central gyrus.

Sensation of pain from the face is served by fibres of the trigeminal nerve which part from their fellows on entering the pons and pass down through the medulla as the descending or spinal trigeminal tract which lies alongside the nucleus of that tract. In its course, fibres pass from the tract to the nucleus where they synapse. The second order neurones cross, then run up through the brain-stem close to the midline as the secondary trigeminal or quintothalamic tract and enter the VPM nucleus of the thalamus. It is probable that there are also projections to the midline reticular formation as in the case of pain fibres from the body.

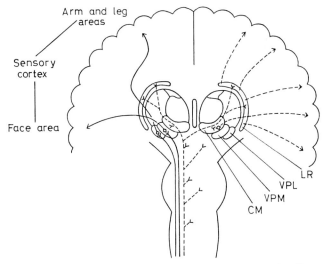

Figure 1.3. Cerebral termination of pain pathways. Specific afferent projections from body and face (spinothalamic and quintothalamic tracts) are indicated as solid lines on the left of the diagram, relaying in nuclei VPL and VPM, and projecting to the post-central sensory cortex. The diffuse spino-reticulo-thalamic pain pathway is displayed as interrupted lines, relaying in the midline thalamic nuclei, centrum medianum (CM) and lateral reticular nucleus (LR), and projecting diffusely to the cerebral cortex (after Bowsher[1], reproduced by courtesy of the editor of 'Brain')

The spinal tract and nucleus of the trigeminal nerve descend into the upper segments of the spinal cord. Fibres are received from the nervus intermedius, glossopharyngeal and vagus nerves, so that the quintothalamic tract transmits impulses from these nerves as well as the trigeminal nerve. Some sensory fibres from the upper three cervical posterior roots synapse with neurones in the spinal trigeminal nucleus, thus permitting referral of pain from the upper head to the neck and vice-versa[11].

Pain appreciation requires the participation of the cortex—not only the primary sensory cortex, but also the frontal and temporal lobes of the brain which add emotional interpretation of the sensation of pain.

As the result of stereotactic operations on the thalamus for the relief of pain, Mark, Ervin and Yakovlev recognize three clinical situations which emphasize our new understanding of pain mechanisms[15].

(1) Profound sensory loss *without* relief of pain. All modalities of sensation are disturbed on clinical examination, but pain is still perceived. Lesion in specific sensory nuclei (VPL and VPM).

(2) No detectable sensory loss *with* relief of pain. Destruction of midline nuclei—intralaminar and parafascicular nuclei.

(3) Little sensory loss or pain relief but ability to ignore pain. Destruction of dorsomedial and anterior thalamic nuclei. This lesion has the same effect as a leucotomy.

Visceral pain

The viscera are insensitive to touching, cutting or pinching, but give rise to the sensation of pain, given an adequate stimulus such as one of the following.

(1) Distension.

(2) Excessive contraction.

(3) Irritation by toxins and chemicals.

True visceral pain must be distinguished from somatic pain caused by the spread of a disease process from the viscus to the surrounding serous membrane or body wall.

Visceral pain is transmitted by the sympathetic nervous system (splanchnic nerves) from the thoracic and abdominal cavities, or the sacral parasympathetic nerves from the pelvis. Certain organic sensations such as hunger, satiety, sense of fullness and nausea appear to be mediated by the vagus nerve, but not the sensation of pain.

Sensory fibres in the gut wall are similar to those in the skin, but are sparser, and smaller in diameter. Free nerve endings in the gut wall and Pacinian corpuscles in the mesentery are the receptors and fibres pass centrally in the splanchnic nerves, traverse the sympathetic ganglia without synapsing, and then enter the posterior roots by way of the white rami communicantes. They have their cell bodies in the posterior root ganglia and their central processes may either:

(*a*) Pass directly upwards in the posterior columns without synapsing (these fibres do not carry pain impulses), or

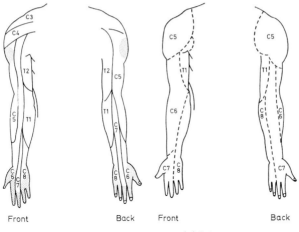

Front   Back   Front   Back

(a) Dermatomes   (b) Sclerotomes

Figure 1.4. Dermatomes and sclerotomes of the upper limb. If one nerve root only is damaged, sensory loss is usually restricted to the dotted areas shown on the left. Paraesthesiae are generally referred to the dermatome and pain to the sclerotome. [Dermatomes, after M.R.C. Memorandum No. 7 'Aids to the Investigation of Peripheral Nerve Injuries'; sclerotomes, after Kellgren[9, 10] (by courtesy of the Editor of Clin. Sci.), and Inman and Saunders[6] (by courtesy of the publishers of J. nerv. ment. Dis.)]

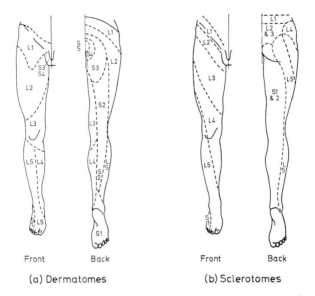

Front   Back   Front   Back

(a) Dermatomes   (b) Sclerotomes

Figure 1.5. Dermatomes and sclerotomes of the lower limb, derived from the same sources as Figure 1.4 (*b*) Synapse in the posterior horns, cross over and ascend in the vicinity of the spinothalamic tracts to the VPL nucleus of the thalamus.

The heart receives sensory fibres from the cardiac nerves, which are connected centrally with T1–4 cord segments.

The splanchnic nerves supply liver, stomach, duodenum, small intestines and kidneys, and run to T6–12 segments of the cord.

The large intestine receives its sympathetic sensory supply via the hypogastric plexus and impulses pass to the T10–L2 segments of the cord.

The pelvic organs are supplied with parasympathetic sensory nerves which enter the spinal cord through the posterior roots of S2–4.

Referred pain

Pain arising from any viscus may appear as though it is arising in any part of the body innervated by the same segments. Recognition of the common types of referred pain is an essential part of clinical diagnosis.

The probable mechanism of referred pain is convergence of somatic and visceral afferent pathways in the central nervous system. This may occur in the posterior horn of the spinal cord or even as high as the VPL nucleus of the thalamus[16]. Thus sensations arising from viscera may be roughly localized by the subject (for example, above or below the umbilicus, in the midline, or in the centre of the chest), or they may be interpreted as coming from various somatic areas.

Kellgren[9, 10] studied the distribution of pain and hyperalgesia which resulted from the injection of hypertonic saline into muscle or interspinous ligaments in man. He found that the areas of referred pain did not correspond exactly to dermatomes described by Foerster but appeared to be projected to the deep structures innervated by the same spinal segment as the structure stimulated. Similar human experiments were carried out by Inman and Saunders who reached the same conclusion as Kellgren and designated the segmental areas of skeletal innervation as 'sclerotomes'[6]. Each dermatome overlies a limited area of the corresponding sclerotome. This concept is illustrated in *Figures 1.4 and 1.5*, which are a composite of those contained in the papers mentioned. The clinical application of these studies is particularly useful in dealing with cases of compression of nerve roots, where pain may be referred diffusely to deep structures approximating to the sclerotome, whereas paraesthesiae are referred precisely to the appropriate dermatome. There is some individual variation in areas of pain reference and spread may occur to adjacent segments in a fashion which is not always predictable.

Phenomena associated with pain

When a painful stimulus is applied to the foot of an experimental animal, the whole limb flexes and the opposite hindlimb extends. These movements, obviously of benefit for protection of the animal, are brought about by multisynaptic reflexes which involve a number of spinal cord segments—the flexor reflex and the crossed extensor response (*Figure 1.6*).

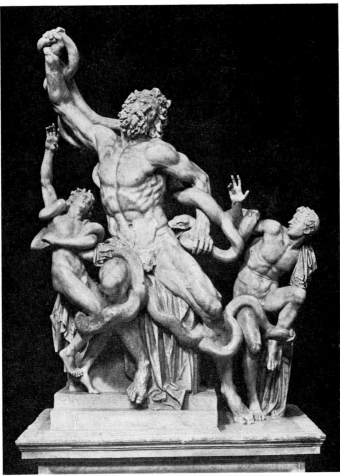

Figure 1.6. Flexor response to a nocuous stimulus, in this instance a sea snake, applied to the lower limb. Weight is supported by the crossed extensor response in the opposite leg (Photograph of 'Laocoön and his sons' by permission of Fratelli Alinari, Florence)

Visceral pain can also cause skeletal muscular contraction, and if the painful stimuli are continued, then muscle contraction is sustained in the form of spasm. This is brought about by polysynaptic reflexes at the segmental level. Thus the anterior abdominal muscles may become rigid over an inflamed viscus, or the whole abdominal wall may be 'board-like' in conditions of general peritoneal inflammation, for example, after rupture of a peptic ulcer. When pain is severe, arms and legs may assume an attitude of flexion.

A similar reflex contraction, this time of extensor muscles of the trunk, may be seen in irritation of the meninges. In extreme cases, a general attitude of extension occurs—neck, trunk and limbs—leading to bowing of the trunk backwards (opisthotonus). More commonly, rigidity of the neck can be felt on attempted flexion, and if the hip is flexed at an angle of 90 degrees to the trunk, the leg cannot be fully extended at the knee (Kernig's sign).

Reflex muscle spasm is often seen around an inflamed joint or in paravertebral muscles when the spine, the vertebrae or the discs between them, are diseased, such contraction having the effect of 'physiological splinting'.

Another common accompaniment of pain is hyperaesthesia of skin areas sharing the same segmental area as the inflamed viscus. This can be abolished by infiltration of the affected area by a local anaesthesic agent, even though pain is still referred to the area. Segmental hyperaesthesia may also occur in disease of the nervous system itself when the nerve roots or posterior root entry zones are affected, for example, the root pains of herpes zoster or girdle pains of myelitis.

Severe pain may produce generalized autonomic disturbance— nausea and vomiting, bradycardia, cutaneous vasoconstriction and lowering of blood pressure with faintness and sweating.

COMMON PATTERNS OF PAIN

Inflammation of skin, muscles or joints
Pain is induced by swelling of the tissues with resulting deformity of pain receptors. Vascular dilatation and oedema are commonly present so that pulsation of the capillaries gives a throbbing quality to the pain. Pain is relieved by placing the affected part in the 'position of rest', that is, the position in which ligaments are relaxed and the tension of interstitial fluid is least, and by elevating the part if it is swollen.

Headache
Headache is caused by the following conditions.

(1) Dilatation or displacement of the *intra*cranial vessels, for example, by drugs or toxins which cause the arteries to dilate, or by a tumour or abscess which stretches the vessels.

(2) Dilatation of the *extra*cranial (scalp) vessels, for example, in migraine.

(3) Irritation of the meninges, for example, meningitis and subarachnoid haemorrhage.

(4) Direct compression of the trigeminal nerve, nervus intermedius (the sensory component of the facial nerve), glossopharyngeal or vagus nerves.

(5) Referred pains from disorders of the eyes, sinuses, teeth or upper cervical spine.

(6) Chronic contraction of the scalp muscles in states of nervous tension.

Cardiac pain
Pain is initiated by ischaemia of cardiac muscle, and is therefore liable to appear when the following circumstances apply.

(1) The filling pressure of the coronary arteries is low (for instance, atheroma of the vessels).

(2) The oxygen-carrying capacity of the blood is diminished (as in severe anaemia).

(3) The heart is doing extra work (for instance, when the patient is walking up a hill).

The pain is characteristically 'pressing' or 'constricting' in nature, and extends across the chest. It may be referred down either arm, most commonly the left, and usually down the inner side of the arm to the elbow (T1–2 segments). It may occasionally extend up the neck to the jaw or down to the upper abdomen.

Cardiac pain may be stimulated by the following conditions.

(1) Dissecting aneurysm of the aorta.

(2) Spasm of the oesophagus, for instance, in hiatus hernia.

(3) States of nervous tension when there is chronic contraction of the muscles of the chest wall. In such cases the pain is persistent, and not clearly related to exertion, and is usually localized by the patient just under the left breast—'over the heart'.

Pleuritic pain
Pain from the inflamed pleura is aggravated by respiratory movement and usually can be accurately localized. If the diaphragmatic pleura is involved in its central part, where the innervation is from the phrenic nerve (C3, 4, 5), pain may be referred to the shoulder. If

the peripheral part of the diaphragm is affected, where the innervation is from the intercostal nerves, pain is referred to the upper abdomen in the distribution of these nerves.

Gastro-intestinal tract pain

Peptic ulcer

The pain of peptic ulcer depends on many factors—inflammatory oedema of tissue around the ulcer, sensitizing nerve endings; contraction of the stomach; the action of hydrochloric acid and other pain-producing substances on the ulcer base[8]. The pain is related to meals, frequently waking the patient at night or coming on at other times when the stomach is empty. It is eased by the taking of food, alkalis, or drugs which diminish the contraction of the stomach. Pain is usually felt in the epigastrium.

If an ulcer has eroded through into the pancreas, or in other forms of pancreatic disease, pain is felt in the back as well as in the epigastrium.

Gall bladder disease

Distension of the gall bladder and biliary tracts results in pain referred to the right hypochondrium and back (T7–9 segments). If the overlying parietal peritoneum is involved, cutaneous hyperaesthesia may be demonstrated in the T7–9 segments. If the diaphragm is irritated by the extension of gall bladder disease, subphrenic abscess, or blood in the peritoneal cavity, pain may be referred to the shoulder, as in the case of diaphragmatic pleurisy.

Bowel

Excessive contraction of the bowel gives rise to a pain which waxes and wanes with the peristaltic waves of the gut (colic). It is poorly localized to the midline above or below the umbilicus. If the parietal peritoneum is affected, for example, in the case of appendicitis, localized pain, tenderness and muscle rigidity may be found over the inflamed area.

Renal tract pain

Afferent fibres from the kidney enter the spinal cord through the tenth to twelfth thoracic nerve roots. Pain from the ureter reaches the cord in the first lumbar segment. Hence disease of the kidney itself gives rise to pain in the back approximately overlying the affected kidney, but when the ureter is in strong contraction, as, for instance, during the passage of a calculus, pain is referred down the L1 segment to the right iliac fossa, groin and testicle on the affected side.

Pain fibres from the bladder are transmitted through the second, third and fourth sacral nerves. Pain from the trigone of the bladder (for example, from a stone in the bladder) may be referred to the tip of the penis. The lower intercostal nerves and first lumbar nerves innervate the peritoneal covering of the bladder.

Ischaemic muscle pain

Muscle pain provoked by exertion, known as intermittent claudication, is caused by an inadequate blood supply allowing accumulation of metabolites.

Pain from disease of the nervous system

Peripheral nerve lesions

Some forms of peripheral neuritis, such as those caused by deficiency of thiamine or vitamin B_{12}, alcoholism and diabetes, are associated with pain and tenderness in the muscles.

Injury to peripheral nerves, particularly the median or sciatic nerves, may give rise to a peculiarly unpleasant burning pain which is known as causalgia. Classical causalgia is characterized by diffuse pain, radiating from the distribution of the affected nerve, and which is aggravated by any contact with the affected area. It is associated with trophic changes in the skin and nails, and is often relieved by sympathectomy. Less severe forms of causalgic pain are seen quite often. Compression of the median nerve in the carpal tunnel, for example, may be responsible for the patient awakening in the night with a diffuse ache, extending above the median nerve distribution to the elbow, or sometimes the shoulder, associated with numbness of the thumb and fingers. It is relieved by moving the limb about but may recur later in the night when the patient is again sleeping.

After amputation of a limb, a diffuse pain may be experienced in the non-existent arm or leg, a condition known as 'phantom limb'. I remember a patient who, after an abdomino-perineal resection of rectum and anus, was plagued by pain in a phantom anus. The mechanism of phantom and causalgic pains is unknown, but is probably the misinterpretation by the nervous system of a disordered pattern of impulses arising in the damaged nerves.

Posterior root lesions

When a posterior root is inflamed or compressed, pain is referred to the sclerotome and paraesthesiae to the appropriate dermatome. For example, in brachial radiculitis involving the fifth and sixth cervical nerve roots, the shoulder may be the site of diffuse pain, while tingling is felt in the thumb and index finger. When the first sacral segment is

15

compressed, pain radiates to the buttock and down the back of the leg as a classical 'sciatica', but paraesthesiae are felt in the sole of the foot. If the fifth lumbar segment is involved, the radiation of pain may be much the same, but paraesthesiae are felt on the dorsum of the foot and the outer side of the calf. Root pain is commonly made worse by bending and any manoeuvre which increases the pressure of CSF in the spinal subarachnoid space such as coughing, sneezing or straining. In the case of lumbar disc lesions, pain is often referred to the groin as well, because the anterior surface of each disc is supplied by a nerve plexus derived chiefly from the first lumbar nerve root.

Herpes zoster causes pain of segmental distribution by direct involvement of the posterior root ganglion. Pain may persist in some individuals after the rash has disappeared. Post-herpetic neuralgia may have the diffuse burning quality of causalgia, probably for the same reason, and is commonly associated with a depressive state.

With chronic syphilitic inflammation of the posterior root ganglion (tabes dorsalis) or with degenerative changes (diabetic myelopathy, or hereditary sensory radicular neuropathy), sharp jabbing pains are felt in the limbs as though they were being stabbed with a knife. These are known as 'lightning pains' and are thought to be caused by spontaneous synchronous discharges of the cells in the posterior root ganglion or its central connexions, analogous to the discharge of motor cells in myoclonic epilepsy.

From spinal cord and brain-stem

Damage to the spinothalamic tracts at any level may initiate a burning pain in the appropriate half of the body below the point at which the tracts are affected. Severe visceral pain of central origin may occur in tabes dorsalis and simulate intestinal obstruction or other abdominal catastrophes. The fifth, ninth and tenth cranial nerves may fire off sensory impulses spontaneously, causing sudden intense pain of brief duration, referred to the sensory distribution of those nerves and commonly precipitated by a stimulus in the appropriate area. Trigeminal and glossopharyngeal neuralgia resemble 'lightning pain' in that the pain is momentary, severe and often repetitive. The vagus nerve also participates in glossopharyngeal neuralgia so that pain is referred to the ear as well as the throat.

From thalamus and cerebral cortex

A thalamic lesion may give rise to an unpleasant diffuse pain similar in quality to that of causalgia, and is evoked similarly by any slight stimulus—hyperpathia or 'thalamic pain'. The sensation of pain may rarely form part of a focal epileptic seizure, when it arises in the sensory cortex.

Pain syndromes of obscure origin

There are many odd pains which are not clearly understood. Some are 'normal pains' in that they are part of the experience of many normal people. The hypochondrial pain or 'stitch' appearing occasionally on exertion is a case in point.

One fairly common pain which receives little space in standard textbooks is 'proctalgia fugax'. This is a paroxysmal pain, felt deeply within the anal canal, which may recur at intervals of weeks, months or years. The condition tends to run in families and has a benign prognosis. A bout of pain may be precipitated by a bowel action or may follow sexual intercourse. During the attack, which lasts from minutes up to an hour, the internal sphincter and levatores ani are in spasm. The pain may be associated with priapism, suggesting that the second and third sacral segments of the spinal cord are in a state of hyperactivity. The pain may be relieved partly by the passage of urine or flatus, by eating or drinking, by lying down, or by suprapubic massage, when it subsides gradually.

Pain associated with states of anxiety or depression

The reaction of a patient to pain may be so biased by affective changes as to make a major disability of a minor symptom.

Some forms of pain may be brought about by excessive muscle contraction associated with nervous tension. Thus, tension headache and atypical facial pains result from over-activity of the scalp and facial muscles in patients who are in the habit of frowning or clenching the jaw. Pain in the neck, back or coccygeal region may arise from contraction of paravertebral muscles. The pain over the praecordium or inframammary pain typical of anxiety states is probably brought about by contraction of intercostal muscles. Certain painful syndromes such as migraine, indigestion and 'spastic colon' are more commonly seen in tense individuals, but the mechanism is indirect and not well understood.

Hysteria

A patient with an hysterical personality will over-react to pain, but pain is not usually a symptom of hysteria. I recollect a patient threatening to jump out of a window because of a pain in her bottom. An eminent surgeon who had examined her several days previously without finding any abnormality thought her to be 'hysterical'. Looking at her bottom again revealed that a large ischio-rectal abscess had developed.

17

Hypochondria

A morbid preoccupation with bodily functions may lead to the interpretation of a any mildly abnormal sensation as pain. This may also be a symptom of depressive illness.

Indifference or insensitivity to pain

Congenital analgesia has been reported in association with a variety of defects of the autonomic nervous system[2].

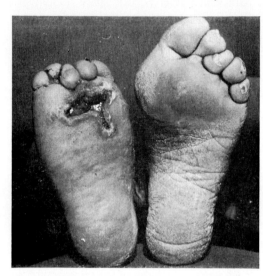

Figure 1.7. Trophic changes in the feet in a patient with analgesia of the legs resulting from hereditary sensory radicular neuropathy. The toes of the right foot are shortened and deformed and there is a perforating ulcer on the sole

Indifference to pain may be encountered rarely as a congenital anomaly, sometimes associated with mental defect, as well as in postencephalitic and hysterical patients. Evoked cortical potentials are of normal amplitude in patients with congenital indifference to pain and hysterical hemianaesthesia.

Pain pathways may be destroyed by disorders such as syringomyelia, Hansen's disease, diabetic neuropathy or hereditary sensory radicular neuropathy. Loss of protective reflexes may lead to degenerative arthritis (Charcot's joints) and trophic lesions of hands or feet (*Figure 1.7*).

CLINICAL HISTORY TAKING IN RELATION TO PAIN

The nature of pain experienced by a patient should be assessed as fully as possible at the initial interview. An adequate first assessment may provide the diagnosis from history alone. It will at least enable one to formulate a rational differential diagnosis and possibly avoid many unnecessary investigations. As the interview progresses, an idea of the patient's intelligence, emotional state and reaction to the pain can be gained and give a lead to questioning about any personal problems which might bias the reaction to pain.

The information to be recorded concerning any pain comprises the following.

Site and radiation.

Quality.

Frequency of recurrence, and duration.

Time and mode of onset.

Associated symptoms, such as nausea, vomiting, sweating.

Precipitating factors, such as breathing, coughing, exertion, hunger, emotional disturbances, micturition, or postures of neck, trunk and limbs.

Relieving factors, such as bodily postures, rest, the taking of food, the application of heat or cold and any drugs which may have been administered.

The exact questions which will be asked of the patient are guided of course by the site of the pain and the thoughts in one's mind about the possible cause of the pain.

THE INTERPRETATION OF SENSORY SYMPTOMS AND SIGNS

At the conclusion of the history the physician should have reached a tentative conclusion about the site of origin of the patients' symptoms so that the physical examination may proceed to test this hypothesis systematically. The distribution of pain and paraesthesiae will suggest whether one or more peripheral nerves or spinal nerve roots are at fault, or whether the symptoms are arising from spinal cord, brain-stem or cerebral hemispheres. Paraesthesiae or numbness in both feet may indicate peripheral neuritis or a spinal cord lesion, but if the sensations spread above the knees the odds swing to a spinal cord disturbance, and if the sensations spread upwards to a level on the trunk, the diagnosis of spinal cord disease is no longer in doubt and a compressing lesion must be promptly excluded. If both hands as well as the feet are involved by paraesthesiae, then the cause must be either a peripheral neuropathy or a lesion of the upper cervical cord or brain-stem. The level of spinal cord involvement may be indicated by a band sensation or a strip of hyperaesthesia on the trunk; Lhermitte's sign indicates a lesion in the cervical part of the spinal cord.

Unilateral paraesthesiae arise from the spinal cord when an intrinsic disorder such as multiple sclerosis, angioma or glioma damages one half selectively, in which case pain and temperature

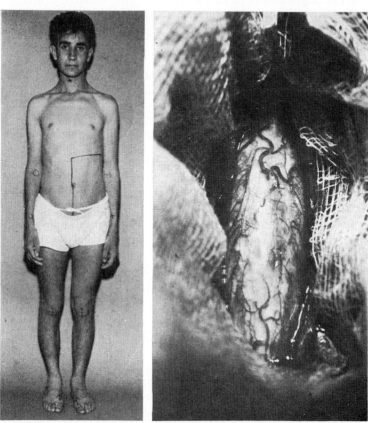

Figure 1.8. Sensory changes with an intramedullary lesion. (a) Sensory loss to pinprick and temperature below the seventh thoracic segmental level on the left side of the body produced by an angioma of the spinal cord in the lower cervical region. Biceps and radial jerks were abolished on the right side and signs of an upper motor neurone lesion were present in both lower limbs; (b) Photograph of the lower cervical spinal cord taken at operation (reproduced by courtesy of Dr. A. Gonski)

sensation will be impaired on the opposite side below the level of the lesion (*Figure 1.8*). There may also be signs of involvement of the pyramidal tract and posterior columns on the same side as the lesion (Brown–Séquard syndrome), or long tracts may be compressed bilaterally. More commonly, unilateral paraesthesiae indicate a disturbance of the brain-stem or one cerebral hemisphere. When one side of the face is involved with the opposite side of the body, the source is clearly in the brain-stem.

Once the distribution of sensory symptoms is established, then the examiner can adapt his sensory examination accordingly. If paraesthesiae are felt in hands and feet, he may begin by asking the patient to contrast the sensation felt in the proximal and distal parts of the limb to see if there is any diminution in sensation peripherally. If there is, then the transition from impaired to normal sensation is mapped rapidly for each limb. Once this is done, the sensation in the proximal part of the limb is contrasted with that on the trunk and face to ensure that there is not a second level of sensory change. If this is not done, the gradation of sensation from the limbs may be interpreted as indicating a peripheral neuropathy, while a clear-cut change at a higher level, for example, between upper cervical segments and the trigeminal area, which points to a lesion near the foramen magnum, may be missed.

If the lower limbs only are involved, then a sensory level on the trunk must be sought carefully, moving from the area of sensory disturbance to that of normal sensation so that the transition may be felt more clearly by the patient. A pin drawn lightly upwards over the trunk may demonstrate a band of hyperaesthesia.

If paraesthesiae are unilateral, sensory examination is concentrated on comparison of the two sides of the body. If abnormal sensations are confined to part of one limb, then the comparison of sensation proceeds from the affected area outwards to delineate it clearly in terms of the peripheral nerves or spinal segments affected.

This procedure seems obvious and logical but is often neglected. A formal sensory examination performed systematically without due regard for the clinical history may lead to the significant disturbance being submerged beneath a contour map of irrelevant artefacts produced by fatigue of both examiner and patient.

PRINCIPLES OF MANAGEMENT OF PAINFUL SYNDROMES

Understanding of the pathophysiology of pain is essential to management as well as diagnosis. A patient who takes aspirin to relieve the pain of peptic ulcer does not assist the healing process.

Pain which is caused by displacement of anatomical structures is relieved by restoration of the normal anatomy. The aspiration of an abscess relieves the tension on pain receptors and the removal of a

21

cerebral tumour relieves headache by permitting pain-sensitive intracranial vessels to return to their normal position. Headache which is caused by dilatation of intracranial vessels can be relieved experimentally by increasing cerebrospinal fluid pressure, whereas headache caused by obstruction to the CSF pathways can be relieved only by reducing intracranial pressure, either by removing the obstruction or by draining the ventricular system.

Extracranial vascular headache, such as migraine, can be relieved by compression of the dilated scalp arteries, and is aborted in most instances by the use of vasoconstrictor agents like ergotamine tartrate. Muscle contraction (tension) headache, by way of contrast, is associated with constriction of extracranial vessels and may be relieved, temporarily at least, by local heat or vasodilator substances like nicotinic acid or alcohol. Vasodilator drugs may also be useful in other ischaemic pain such as angina pectoris and intermittent claudication, although the latter usually requires the surgical removal of mechanical obstruction to blood flow.

Pain from excessive contraction of smooth muscle in the renal, biliary or gastrointestinal tract may respond to anticholinergic agents.

Splinting an inflamed limb, or strapping one side of the chest affected by pleurisy are age-old methods of relieving pain by rest. Elevation of an inflamed part will reduce the throbbing pain evoked by vascular congestion. The application of heat or cold, counter-irritation of the appropriate skin segments by rubbing, the use of liniments, vibration, or massage of affected muscles, are often helpful in the relief of pain. These simple measures tend to be forgotten and potent analgesic drugs used in their stead.

Where back pain is the result of nerve root compression by a degenerated lumbar disc, extension exercises are advised to build up the back muscles so as to provide an internal brace, which is much more effective than any externally applied brace. Pain can often be relieved by lumbar traction before attempting extension exercises, and the patient can apply traction himself by hanging by the hands from a horizontal bar or the lintel of an old-style doorway, so that the weight of the pelvis and legs is applied to stretch the lumbar spine. A simple manipulation of the lumbo-sacral spine will often relieve the pain of an acute lumbar disc lesion. With the patient lying prone, one hand is placed firmly over the iliac crest and sacrum, while the leg of the same side is forcibly extended and adducted so as to apply a rotational strain to the lumbo-sacral joint (*Figure 1.9*). The procedure is then repeated with the other leg, the rotation being in the reverse direction.

Cervical traction is helpful in patients with cervical spondylosis to relieve pain in the neck, shoulders and arms. It is advisable for this to be done by a trained physiotherapist. Manipulation of the neck is not generally advisable because of the danger of precipitating

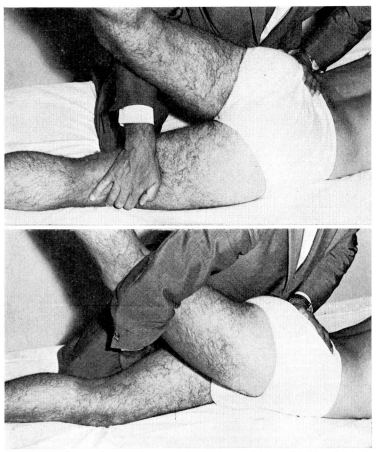

Figure 1.9. Diagonal manipulation of the lumbosacral joint. (a) The clinician's left hand presses firmly over the left side of the sacrum and adjacent iliac crest, while the left thigh is extended and adducted at the hip joint; (b) the pressure is then transferred to the right side while the right thigh is extended and adducted. It should be noted that the procedure is unsuitable for those patients whose pain is made much worse by a preliminary gentle extension of the leg

compression of the cervical spinal cord with resulting quadriparesis.

Pains caused by paroxysmal and synchronous neuronal discharge, like trigeminal neuralgia and lightning pains, usually respond well to

23

anticonvulsant medication, carbamazepine (Tegretol) being the most effective drug.

Certain pains are associated with, and perhaps perpetuated by, a depressive state. Many cases of chronic tension headache, atypical facial pain, post-herpetic neuralgia, backache and coccydynia respond to antidepressant drugs. Amitriptyline (Tryptanol, Tryptizol, Larozyl, Elavil) and imipramine (Tofranil) may produce striking amelioration of chronic tension headache[12]. Tranquillizing agents like chlordiazepoxide (Librium) and diazepam (Valium) may have a similar beneficial effect on the tense and anxious patient.

Further advances in the management of pain may be expected with the elucidation of the part played by chemical substances such as serotonin and bradykinin in provoking pain. It has recently been shown that aspirin may relieve pain by acting as an antagonist to the action of bradykinin on sensory receptors[14]. It may well be that chemical agents are developed in the future to block specifically the actions of certain substances at certain sites. It is known that local anaesthetic agents such as procaine act non-specifically by blocking small nerve fibres concerned with pain perception before large fibres are affected.

Finally, when pain can no longer be relieved by physiological or pharmacological measures, some destructive operation on pain pathways may have to be undertaken. When the section of peripheral nerves or posterior roots does not relieve pain, anterolateral cordotomy, stereotactic thalamotomy or leucotomy may be necessary. As knowledge of the anatomical and physiological basis of pain advances, such operations are becoming more selective and failures less frequent.

SUMMARY

Normal sensation depends upon the recognition by the central nervous system of a pattern formed by impulses which have been deployed in time and space by their passage along a number of nerve fibres of different calibre. When the pattern of impulses is disorganized or the frequency of impulses is excessive, distorted sensations or pain may be experienced by the patient. Pain is subjective and the threshold to pain may vary according to the emotional state.

The quality and distribution of different sensations enables the clinician to predict their site or origin with reasonable accuracy. Knowledge of dermatomes and sclerotomes is essential in the diagnosis of nerve root irritation or of the segments involved in referred pain.

Pain is generally referred to the sclerotome and paraesthesiae to the dermatome. Pain is often accompanied by segmental hyperaesthesia and reflex muscle contraction. The pattern of pain or paraesthesiae elicited in history-taking guides the clinician in making a selective sensory examination to test the hypothesis suggested by the history.

The management of painful syndromes depends upon an understanding of the pathophysiology of pain, which includes the emotional reaction of the patient. New knowledge of pathways associated with the perception of pain makes it possible to relieve intractable pain without impairing the patient's ability to distinguish between sharp and blunt stimuli.

REFERENCES

[1] Bowsher, D. (1957). 'Termination of the central pain pathway in man: The conscious appreciation of pain.' *Brain* **80**, 606–622
[2] Brown, J. W. and Podosin, R. (1966). 'A syndrome of the neural crest.' *Archs. Neurol.* **15**, 294–301
[3] Calne, D. B. and Pallis, C. A. (1966). 'Vibratory sense: A critical review.' *Brain* **89**, 723–746
[4] Eccles, J. C. (1964). 'The controls of sensory communication to the brain.' *Australas. Ann. Med.* **13**, 102–113
[5] Halliday, A. M. and Wakefield, G. S. (1963). 'Cerebral evoked potentials in patients with dissociated sensory loss.' *J. Neurol. Psychiat.* **26**, 211–219
[6] Inman, V. T. and Saunders, J. B. de C. M. (1944). 'Referred pain from skeletal structures.' *J. nerv. ment. Dis.* **99**, 660–667
[7] Jabbur, S. J. and Towe, A. L. (1961). 'Cortical excitation of neurons in dorsal column nuclei, including an analysis of pathways.' *J. Neurophysiol.* **24**, 499–509
[8] Keele, C. A. and Armstrong, D. (1964). *Substances Producing Pain and Itch.* London; Edward Arnold
[9] Kellgren, J. H. (1939). 'Observations on referred pain arising from muscle.' *Clin. Sci.* **3**, 175–190
[10] Kellgren, J. H. (1939). 'On the distribution of pain arising from deep somatic structures with charts of segmental pain areas.' *Clin. Sci.* **4**, 35–46
[11] Kerr, F. W. L. (1961). 'Trigeminal and cervical volleys.' *Archs. Neurol.* **5**, 171–178
[12] Lance, J. W. and Curran, D. A. (1964). 'Treatment of chronic tension headache.' *Lancet* **1**, 1236–1239
[13] Lele, P. P. and Weddell, G. (1956). 'The relationship between neurohistology and corneal sensibility.' *Brain* **79**, 119–154
[14] Lim, R. K. S., Miller, D. G., Guzman, F., Rodgers, D. W., Rogers, R. W., Wang, S. K., Chao, P. Y. and Shih, T. Y. (1967). 'Pain and analgesia evaluated by the intraperitoneal bradykinin-evoked pain method in man.' *Clin. Pharmac. Ther.* **8**, 521–542
[15] Mark, V. H., Ervin, F. R. and Yakovlev, P. I. (1963). 'Stereotactic Thalamotomy III. The verification of anatomical lesion sites in the human thalamus.' *A.M.A. Archs. Neurol.* **8**, 528–538

[16] McLeod, J. G. (1958). 'The representation of the splanchnic afferent pathways in the thalamus of the cat.' *J. Physiol.* **140,** 462–478

[17] Melzack, R. and Wall, P. D. (1962). 'On the nature of cutaneous sensory mechanisms.' *Brain* **85,** 331–356

[18] Nathan, P. W. and Rice, R. C. (1966). 'The localization of warm stimuli.' *Neurology* **16,** 533–544

[19] Rose, J. E. and Mountcastle, V. B. (1959). 'Touch and kinesthesis.' In *American Physiological Society Handbook of Physiology.* Ed. by J. Field. Sect. 1, Vol. 1, pp. 387–429. Baltimore; Williams and Wilkins

[20] Sinclair, D. C. and Stokes, B. A. R. (1964). 'The production and characteristics of "second pain".' *Brain* **87,** 609–618

[21] Towe, A. L. and Jabbur, S. J. (1961). 'Cortical inhibition of neurons in dorsal column nuclei of cat.' *J. Neurophysiol.* **24,** 488–498

2—Weakness

One of the main concerns of this book is an analysis of the way in which the motor system works and the manner in which its disorders are manifested as physical signs. Before attempting this dissection, it seems logical to discuss the symptom of weakness which brings most patients with motor disorders to their doctor.

There is a lack of precision about the meaning of weakness which must be clarified at the beginning of the clinical history. There are some patients whose complaint of weakness may really mean loss of balance, loss of joint position sense, muscular rigidity, or a whole host of sensory or other disturbances which have no component of paresis. Motor and sensory symptoms may also become confused in the reverse direction so that a patient may speak of his limb feeling numb or dead when he means that he is unable to move it in the normal fashion.

Weakness may imply a subjective sensation of lassitude, fatigue and exhaustion, when it is classified as asthenia. The term weakness may also be used for a progressive failure in the power of muscular contraction with repeated or sustained exertion, in which case it is called myasthenia, and suggests a failure of neuromuscular conduction or a metabolic defect in muscle. Most commonly, weakness means that normal force cannot be exerted by a muscle or group of muscles (paresis) or that part of the body is paralyzed.

The primary source of physical weakness may be in muscle or at one or other level of the nervous system. The clinician determines the probable source by the history of evolution of weakness, whether steadily progressive or intermittent in its temporal pattern, the distribution of muscles affected, and the associated clinical signs. Physical weakness may be simulated by hysteria and the ways in which the two may be distinguished are considered at the end of a general survey of the various causes of weakness.

ASTHENIA

The complaint of feeling generally tired and weak, without any more specific symptoms, is one of the most difficult problems in clinical medicine to assess and manage. Asthenia may be a symptom of anaemia, low cardiac output, an occult neoplasm, an infection or some chronic systemic disease. It may be a symptom of endocrine disease such as underactivity or overactivity of the thyroid or adrenal glands, deficiency in ovarian or testicular function, hypopituitarism or hyperparathyroidism. It may be the result of carbohydrate intolerance with reactionary hypoglycaemia, possibly as an early indication of diabetes mellitus. The association of asthenia with undue drowsiness, akin to narcolepsy, has been described in hypo-glycaemic patients[6]. Hypoglycaemic symptoms may be a feature of liver disease, endocrine disorders and insulin-secreting tumours.

Asthenia is also a common symptom of psychological origin, the severity of the underlying disorder ranging from sheer boredom to profound depression. Accompanying symptoms of anxiety or hysteria, such as faintness, sweating, palpitations and paraesthesiae may resemble those of organic forms of asthenia, particularly hypoglycaemia. The following dialogue poses the problem of asthenia, organic or functional?

> FALSTAFF. and I hear, moreover, his highness is fallen into this same whoreson apoplexy.
>
> CHIEF JUSTICE. Well, heaven mend him! I pray you, let me speak with you.
>
> FALSTAFF. This apoplexy is, as I take it, a kind of lethargy, an't please your lordship; a kind of sleeping in the blood, a whoreson tingling.
>
> CHIEF JUSTICE. What tell you me of it? be it as it is.
>
> FALSTAFF. It hath its original from much grief, from study and perturbation of the brain. I have read the cause of his effects in Galen.
>
> (*King Henry IV, Part II*).

Patients with the asthenic syndrome are often incorrectly diagnosed as having myasthenia gravis and are treated with large doses of anticholinesterase agents. These may produce some subjective benefit by the non-specific stimulant effect of acetylcholine, thus making the distinction from myasthenia gravis more difficult[4, 5].

The diagnosis of myasthenia gravis depends upon the development on exertion of muscular paresis (ptosis, diplopia, dysphagia, difficulty in coughing, or inability to maintain contraction of limb muscles) which is reversed under observation by anticholinesterase drugs.

PARALYSIS OR PARESIS

True muscular weakness is an indication of disorder of the motor system at some point in the chain of control which extends from the cells of the motor cortex to the muscle fibre (*Figure 2.1*).

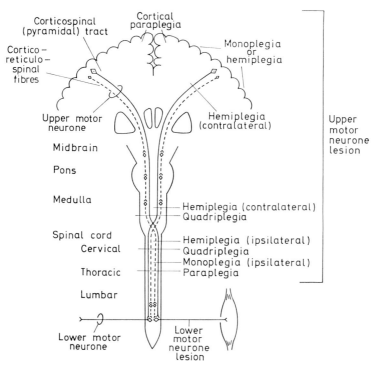

Figure 2.1. Schema of upper and lower motor neurones, showing the levels of the nervous system at which they may be affected and the distribution of weakness which results. The pyramidal tract is shown as being accompanied by a cortico-reticulo-spinal pathway, whose involvement by disease is responsible for the phenomena of spasticity

Pyramidal lesions
A pure pyramidal lesion is rarely seen clinically and is not associated with gross spasticity.

Upper motor neurone lesions

An upper motor neurone lesion is the common clinical syndrome caused by involvement of areas 4 and 6 or their projection pathways, that is, lesions of the pyramidal tract together with closely associated extrapyramidal fibres (*Figure 2.1*). An upper motor neurone lesion results from destruction of motor pathways in cerebral cortex, internal capsule, cerebral peduncles, brain-stem or spinal cord. Here weakness is associated with increased tonic and phasic stretch reflexes (spasticity). Resistance to muscle stretch is encountered on passive movement of a limb and tendon jerks become hyperactive. Commonly, but not invariably, an upper motor neurone lesion is associated with an extensor plantar response. The mechanism of spasticity is discussed in later chapters.

Weakness of upper motor neurone origin affects chiefly the extensor and abductors of the upper limbs, distally more than proximally, and, in contrast, affects flexor groups more than extensors in the lower limbs.

Monoplegia

Weakness may affect one limb only if the appropriate area of the cerebral cortex or its projection pathway is selectively damaged. One arm may become weak after thrombosis of the recurrent branch of the anterior cerebral artery (Heubner's artery) which supplies a part of the internal capsule. One leg may be affected if the anterior cerebral artery thromboses distal to its recurrent branch so that infarction is limited to the 'leg area' of motor cortex. With a cortical monoparesis, there is usually some indication of motor disturbance elsewhere on the same side of the body—a little weakness or lower facial movement, diminution of abdominal reflexes, or minimal weakness of the other limb.

Hemiplegia

The projection pathways from all areas of motor cortex are commonly involved together in brain or brain-stem, leading to contralateral weakness. A lesion of one half of the spinal cord in the upper cervical region can produce an ipsilateral hemiparesis as part of a Brown–Séquard syndrome, but in practice, there is usually some impairment of the opposite side so that the disturbance becomes a quadriparesis.

Hemiparesis may result from compression of the brain by subdural or extradural haematoma or extracerebral tumour such as meningioma. More commonly, hemiparesis is produced by an intrinsic lesion such as cerebral contusion, infarction, haemorrhage or intracerebral tumour.

If, therefore, the commencement of the affection be below the head, such as the membrane of the spinal marrow, the parts which are homonymous and connected with it are paralysed: the right on the right side, and the left on the left side. But if the head be primarily affected on the right side, the left side of the body will be paralysed; and the right, if on the left side. The cause of this is the interchange in the origins of the nerves, for they do not pass along on the same side, the right on the right side, until their terminations; but each of them passes over to the other side from that of its origin, decussating each other in the form of the letter X.

Aretaeus of Cappadocia. c. 150 A.D.

Paraplegia and quadriplegia

Weakness of both legs is usually the result of spinal cord damage, but may occasionally be caused by a cortical lesion involving the upper end of the motor strip bilaterally, such as a parasagittal meningioma or a depressed fracture of the skull. Bilateral damage to the upper motor neurone in the internal capsules, brain-stem or the upper cervical portion of the spinal cord causes a spastic weakness of all four limbs (quadriparesis) or complete paralysis (quadriplegia). Weakness of both legs (paraparesis or paraplegia) results from disruption of the upper motor neurone in the lower cervical or thoracic spinal canal. The lumbar vertebrae contain the conus medullaris and cauda equina, so that any damage in this region produces a lower motor neurone weakness of the legs.

Compression of the spinal cord by vertebral disease (fracture-dislocation, Pott's disease, secondary tumours), disc degeneration, pacchymeningitis or tumours such as neurofibroma or meningioma, must be diagnosed early, since this group of conditions is usually remediable by surgery. Intrinsic lesions of the cord are less tractable, although subacute combined degeneration of the spinal cord may be prevented from progressing by treating vitamin B_{12} deficiency, and recovery from acute episodes of demyelination may be hastened by adrenocorticotrophin. Diabetic, syphilitic or malignant myelopathies are uncommon, but may respond partly to management of the underlying condition. Thrombosis of the anterior spinal artery may be associated with insufficiency of the vertebral arteries from which it takes its origin. Below the cervical region, the vascular supply to the anterior two thirds of spinal cord is derived from the aorta by branches from intercostal and lumbar arteries. For this reason, the vascular supply of the cord suffers in dissecting aneurysm or atherothrombotic disease of the aorta (*Figure 2.2*). Angioma or

31

glioma of the spinal cord may be responsible for progressive para-paresis (*see Figure 1.4*). Syringomyelia or haematomyelia are less common intrinsic lesions in which the sensory changes are usually more evident than paraparesis. Motor neurone disease is the name given to a disorder of unknown aetiology, in which both upper and lower motor neurones degenerate, giving rise to a combination of muscular wasting and fasciculation with increased tendon jerks and extensor plantar responses. There is a hereditary form of spastic paraplegia, which is rare and is unrelated to motor neurone disease.

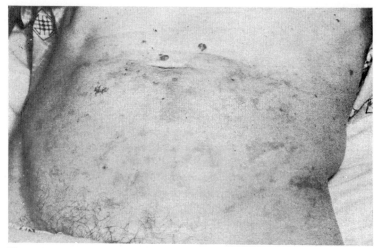

Figure 2.2. Patchy ecchymoses below the umbilicus as a result of embolism from a thrombosis of the aorta. The patient suffered a paraplegia affecting muscles innervated below the ninth thoracic segment

THE LOWER MOTOR NEURONE

Damage to the lower motor neurone at any point from the anterior horn cell to the neuromuscular junction produces a flaccid paralysis with diminution or absence of the deep reflexes and wasting of muscles (*Figure 2.3*).

Muscle fibres, when partly or wholly denervated, may contract spontaneously. This is called fasciculation when a whole motor unit is involved, and this movement is coarse enough to be seen under the skin. When individual muscle fibres are discharging independently, the process is called fibrillation and can be seen only in the tongue, although it can be readily recorded elsewhere by electromyography.

The distribution of lower motor neurone weakness is segmental when the spinal motor neurones, motor roots, or brachial or lumbosacral nerve plexuses are damaged. For example, when the fifth and sixth cervical nerve roots are compressed or inflamed, the scapular muscles, deltoid, biceps and brachioradialis muscles become weak and the biceps and brachioradialis (radial, supinator) tendon

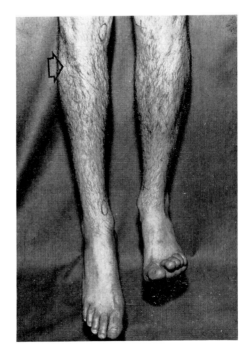

Figure 2.3. Right foot drop from compression of the fourth and fifth lumbar and first sacral motor nerve roots. The anterolateral compartment of the right leg is wasted (arrow) and the right knee and ankle jerks are absent

jerks are abolished. The signs will be the same if the upper cord of the brachial plexus is injured. Distal to the great nerve plexuses of the upper and lower limbs, the contribution from various spinal segments become interwoven in the formation of peripheral nerves. The distribution of weakness from a peripheral nerve lesion must therefore be distinguished from that of the spinal segments of which the nerve is comprised. A case in point is wasting of the small muscles of the hand, which may be caused by a lesion of the first thoracic spinal segment or of the ulnar nerve (*Figure 2.4*). The only two hand muscles which do not receive any motor innervation from the ulnar nerve are the abductor pollicis brevis and opponens pollicis so that they remain intact in ulnar nerve lesions. If these muscles are

33

impaired with the rest, it shows that wasting cannot be explained solely by an ulnar nerve lesion and suggests that the source must be sought proximally in the first thoracic segment.

Anterior horn cells may be damaged by an acute illness such as poliomyelitis, transverse myelitis, or vascular occlusion. They may slowly degenerate in motor neurone disease (or in the rare

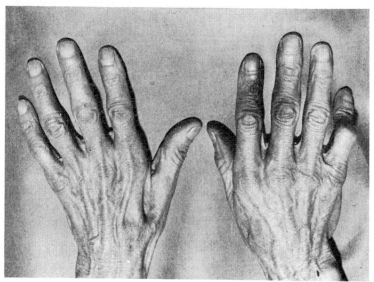

Figure 2.4. Wasting of the small muscles of the hand, seen in a bilateral lesion of the ulnar nerve or the first thoracic spinal segment

diabetic or syphilitic myelopathies). They may be destroyed by tumours within the spinal cord or by the expansion of a tube-like cavity (syringomyelia). The motor roots, after emerging from the spinal cord may be compressed by degenerated intervertebral disc substance, diseased vertebrae or extramedullary tumours. Brachial radiculitis is an acute inflammation of cervical nerve roots, commonly the fifth and sixth, which causes severe pain in the shoulder and upper limb, followed by weakness and wasting of segmental distribution (neuralgic amyotrophy). All motor roots may be involved in Guillain–Barré syndrome, an acute ascending paralysis.

The brachial plexus may be damaged by trauma, tumour or irradiation fibrosis, and its lower cord may be compressed by a cervical rib, by fibrous bands in the thoracic inlet, or by carcinoma of the apex of the lung (Pancoast tumour), with weakness of muscles

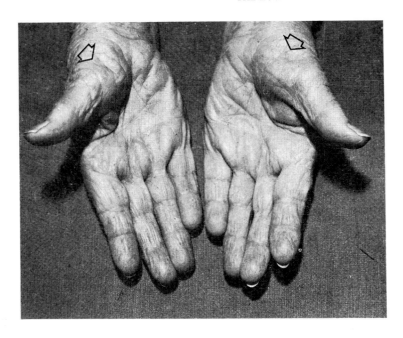

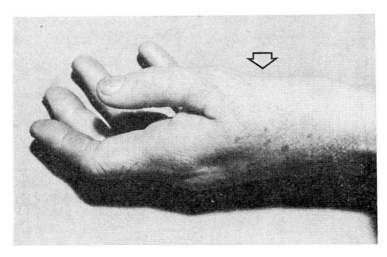

Figure 2.5. Selective wasting of the abductor pollicis brevis bilaterally (arrowed), caused by compression of the median nerves in the carpal tunnels

supplied by the eighth cervical and first thoracic segments. The lumbosacral plexus may be compressed by pelvic tumours.

Individual peripheral nerves may be affected by an anaphylactic process or a chronic inflammation such as leprosy, or they may be compressed at some point in their course. Classical examples are wasting of the hand muscles with an ulnar nerve lesion (*Figure 2.4*), wasting of the abductor pollicis brevis when the median nerve is compressed in the carpal tunnel (*Figure 2.5*), wrist drop from compression of the radial nerve and foot drop from damage to the lateral popliteal nerve. Disorder of a single peripheral nerve is termed mononeuritis, and if more than one peripheral nerve is discretely involved, the condition is called mononeuritis multiplex. All peripheral nerves may be involved together by a wide variety of deficiency, metabolic, toxic and other disorders. The condition is then known as polyneuropathy, polyneuritis or peripheral neuropathy[8]. Either motor or sensory symptoms may predominate and commonly affect the distal parts of the limbs symmetrically.

THE NEUROMUSCULAR JUNCTION

Transmission at the neuromuscular junction depends upon the release of acetylcholine from the synaptic vesicles of terminal nerve branches of motor fibres, which lie partly embedded in the sarcoplasm of the endplate (*Figure 2.6*). In the resting state, miniature endplate potentials are recorded by an electrode close to the synaptic region. These are about 1 per cent of the amplitude of the normal endplate potential produced by impulses in motor nerves and are thought to be caused by the liberation of small packets or quanta of acetylcholine from the presynaptic terminals[1]. The amplitude of miniature potentials is reduced in myasthenia gravis, suggesting that this condition is associated with a failure of synthesis or release of acetylcholine. Repetitive electrical stimulation of a motor nerve in a normal subject does not lead to any fatigue of the neuromuscular junction unless a fast rate of stimulation is maintained. The muscle potential may decline to 50 per cent over a period of 30 seconds when the stimulation frequency reaches 50/second[7]. In disorders of the neuromuscular junction, such as myasthenia gravis, the muscle potential fails progressively with repetitive stimulation but may be restored by the use of anticholinesterase agents which permit the accumulation of acetylcholine in the synaptic cleft between nerve and muscle.

The neuromuscular junction may be paralysed by certain drugs or toxins acting either on the donor surface of the axon terminals or the receptor surface of the muscle endplate (*Figure 2.7*). Hemicholinium impairs synthesis of acetylcholine. Tetanus, botulinus and tick toxins, neomycin and excessive concentrations of magnesium ions prevent the release of acetylcholine, thus blocking transmission

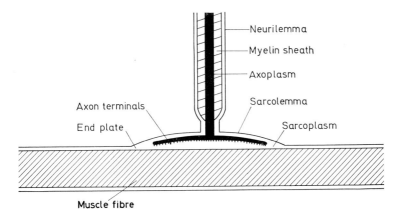

Figure 2.6. Schema of the neuromuscular junction

while the muscle endplate remains polarized (polarization block). Polarization block is also produced by curare or succinylcholine which compete with acetylcholine for receptors on the muscle

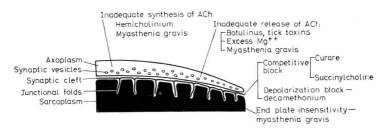

Figure 2.7. Detail of the neuromuscular junction showing factors which affect transmission

endplate. Decamethonium, on the other hand, prevents effective neuromuscular transmission by depolarizing the muscle endplate, the paralysis therefore being called depolarization block.

Progressive failure of neuromuscular transmission is accompanied by fatigue of muscle contraction and paresis (myasthenia). The best known myasthenic state is myasthenia gravis, which is thought to

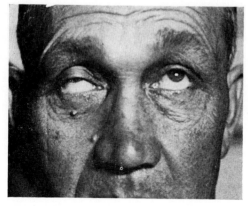

Figure 2.8. Right ptosis in a patient with myasthenia gravis. The ptosis disappeared completely after the intravenous injection of edrophonium

be an autoimmune process, interfering with the synthesis or release of acetylcholine. There remains some doubt as to whether the post-synaptic membrane is also affected[2].

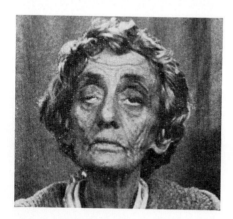

Figure 2.9. Advanced myasthenia gravis with muscular wasting. Paresis persists in spite of anticholinesterase agents

The muscular paresis which is observed in myasthenic patients after exertion may be reversed for a few minutes by the intravenous injection of edrophonium 10 mg, or for several hours by neostigmine or pyridostigmine. These anticholinesterase agents are used as a

1diagnostic test; neostigmine and pyridostigmine are employed in treatment. Increasing the retention of potassium by giving supplements of potassium together with spironolactone (Aldactone-A) is a useful adjuvant method of treatment. In the advanced state of myasthenia gravis, an irreversible deficit may be associated with muscular wasting (*Figure 2.9*).

The myasthenic state may occasionally appear as a symptom of polymyositis, polyneuritis or motor neurone disease, and has also been reported after poliomyelitis, presumably because axon terminals are damaged in these conditions. A variation on the theme of myasthenia has been recognized in the neuromyopathy associated with carcinoma of the lung. In this condition, the muscle action potential evoked by a single nerve stimulus is smaller than normal, but the amplitude increases during repetitive stimulation at 10–200/second. Calcium and guanidine, which increase the amount of acetylcholine released by the nerve impulse, are more effective than the use of anticholinesterase agents in the carcinomatous myasthenic syndrome[3].

MUSCLE

Disorders of muscle (myopathies) may cause weakness or paralysis in the presence of an intact nervous system. Myopathic weakness generally affects proximal rather than distal muscles and the face is commonly involved. Muscle tone and deep reflexes are diminished in proportion to muscle weakness and not impaired selectively as they may be in peripheral neuropathies. The many forms of muscle disease are discussed in a volume edited by Walton[9]. A number of categories may be distinguished.

The muscular dystrophies
Muscular dystrophies form a group of genetically determined disorders in which certain muscles become progressively weaker and wasted. In some varieties, the weakness remains limited to the face or the face and limb girdles, so that life span may be virtually normal (*Figure 2.10*). In Duchenne dystrophy, weakness continues to advance and causes death of the patient before adult life. While most limb and trunk muscles waste away, the calf muscles are larger than normal in Duchenne dystrophy, although they later become weak and infiltrated with fat (pseudohypertrophy) (*Figure 2.11*). In other forms of muscular dystrophy, there is difficulty in relaxing muscles once they are contracted (myotonia). This may be found as an isolated congenital defect (myotonia congenita) or as a part of a complex of genetic defects known as dystrophia myotonica.

39

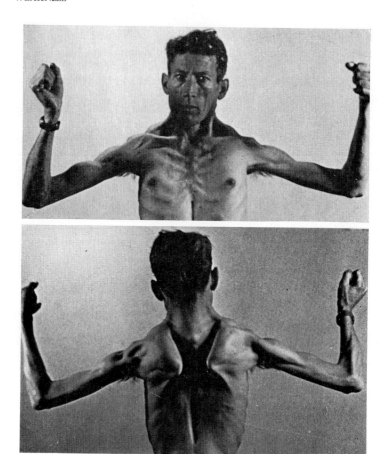

Figure 2.10. Wasting of the upper limb girdle in facio-scapulo-humeral muscular dystrophy

Polymyositis

Polymyositis is an inflammatory reaction in muscle of unknown aetiology which causes weakness of proximal muscles. There may be no obvious signs of inflammation such as tenderness or swelling, redness and warmth in the overlying skin to indicate its nature,and diagnosis may have to rely upon electromyography and muscle biopsy. Polymyositis may be associated with other presumably autoimmune diseases involving the skin or collagen tissue.

40

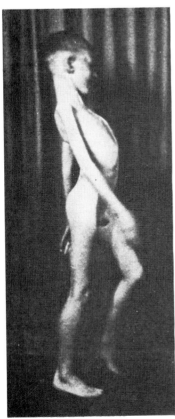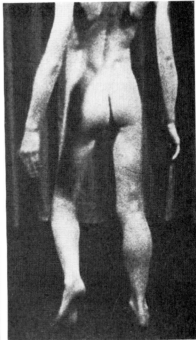

Figure 2.11. Lordotic gait in Duchenne muscular dystrophy. The hypertrophic calves contrast with the wasting of muscles elsewhere

Secondary myopathies

Proximal muscular weakness is a feature of many endocrine disorders, seen commonly in thyrotoxicosis and excessive adrenal cortical activity (Cushing's syndrome). Myopathy may also be secondary to chronic alcoholism or to the presence of a carcinoma, particularly of the lung, which may not give rise to other symptoms at a stage when it produces muscular weakness. The secondary myopathies improve when the underlying condition is controlled.

Metabolic abnormalities

Changes in potassium balance may induce profound generalized weakness or even complete paralysis. Potassium may be lost from the body by vomiting, diarrhoea or urinary excretion. Hypokal-aemia may reach dangerous levels in the recovery phase of diabetic coma, in potassium-losing nephropathy, aldosteronism, the long-continued use of diuretic agents or adrenal corticosteroids.

There are also familial forms of periodic paralysis, the most common of which is associated with a low serum potassium level.

A rare genetic metabolic disorder, McArdle's syndrome, causes fatigue and cramps on exertion with contracture of the muscle if exercise continues. The syndrome is caused by an absence of muscle phosphorylase so that the metabolism of glycogen is blocked.

HYSTERICAL WEAKNESS

The patient who complains of weakness, has signs of weakness and yet has no organic neuromuscular disorder may be consciously simulating disability or may have repressed this fact so that belief in the disability is genuine. Malingering shades almost imperceptibly into the condition of conversion hysteria, where the patient tries to convince the physician because he has convinced himself. Inade-quacy of intelligence, education and personality combine with suggestibility to provide the basis for hysteria. The precipitation of apparently organic manifestations is usually the result of real or imagined wrongs, or an escape from some tedious, unpleasant or threatening life situation. The presentation may be that of weakness, but sensory loss, blindness, loss of vision and loss of memory for long periods of automatic behaviour (hysterical fugues) are not uncommon. The recognition of hysterical weakness and its manage-ment can provide examples of instant cures at the bedside, although the long-term outlook is uncertain if the underlying causes remain unaltered.

Suspicion of hysterical weakness may be aroused during history-taking by an unusual pattern of onset and the impression may be heightened by a curious faraway look in the patient's eye and by his or her emotional detachment from the events being related. The element of drama may embellish the story and histrionic gestures accompany attempts to stand or walk (*Figure 2.12*). The distribution of weakness may not fit into any organic pattern but, more impor-tant, there are two characteristics of hysterical weakness which usually enable a diagnosis to be made. One is the contraction of muscles antagonistic to those being tested, in order to provide a braking action on the force exerted and thus give the impression of weakness to the examiner. For example, the tendons on the instep and dorsum of the foot are seen to stand out when plantarflexors

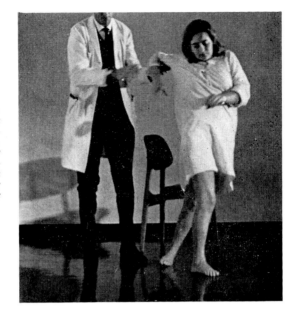

Figure 2.12. Abnormal gait in a patient with hysterical weakness. The patient adopts a variety of histrionic postures which do not resemble those of any organic disease

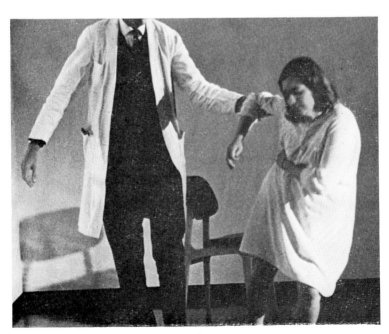

43

are being tested or the hamstrings tendons are felt to become taut while quadriceps power is examined. The simultaneous contraction of agonist and antagonist is observed only in hysteria or dystonia, and the latter can be distinguished on other grounds, discussed in later chapters. The second characteristic of hysterical weakness is the absence of counter pressure which is normally exerted during maximal contraction. This can be observed most easily in the lower limbs while hip flexion is being tested. Normally, a hand placed

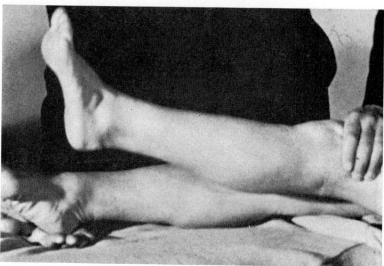

Figure 2.13. Lack of counter-pressure by the hip extensors of the opposite leg when the power of hip flexion is being tested (Hoover's sign). In this illustration of a patient with hysterical paralysis, the heel is not even touching the examiner's hand

under one heel feels strong counter pressure when the opposite leg is elevated and maintained in position against an examiner's weight applied above the knee. In hysterical weakness, only a small proportion of the power of hip extensors is exerted in counter-pressure (Hoover's sign). In some instances the heel may actually ride above the examiner's hand (*Figure 2.13*).

TRANSIENT PARALYSIS

Brief episodes of hemiparesis may be an expression of recurrent oedema in the neighbourhood of a progressive cerebral lesion such as cerebral tumour, or a symptom of intermittent cerebral vascular insufficiency. If ischaemia in the territory of one internal carotid artery is responsible, the hemiparesis is contralateral and may be associated with aphasia, paraesthesiae and other symptoms of cortical origin, or with transient dimness of vision on the side of the stenosed artery, since the ophthalmic artery arises from the internal carotid artery. If the basilar artery is at fault, the side of hemiplegia may vary from episode to episode or both sides of the body may become weak together.

There are a number of possible causes of falling attacks in which the antigravity muscles are suddenly deprived of function by failure of the descending motor pathways.

(1) Functional interruption of descending motor pathways by ischaemia of the brain-stem (vertebrobasilar insufficiency). The motor tracts originating in the brain-stem (vestibulospinal and reticulospinal tracts) cease functioning and a sudden weakness and loss of posture ensues.

(2) Falling attacks of petit mal and myoclonus. The motor cortex, reticular formation and descending motor pathways are temporarily inactivated by an epileptic process.

(3) Cataplexy. Here a more gradual loss of posture follows laughing or other expression of emotion, caused by inhibition of descending reticulospinal pathways. Cataplexy is often associated with narcolepsy or 'forced sleep' which is caused by a similar wave of inhibition, this time affecting the ascending reticulospinal pathways. Cataplexy is an extension of the familiar sensation called 'weak with laughter'.

More prolonged episodes of recurrent paralysis are produced by metabolic disorders such as hypokalaemia.

The course of weakness in multiple sclerosis is commonly one of relapsing and remitting over months or years, although in a minority of patients the disorder progresses steadily.

THE CLINICAL APPROACH TO THE PROBLEM OF WEAKNESS

The nature of the complaint of weakness unfolds as history-taking progresses. The mental and emotional state of the patient is particularly relevant when the sensation of weakness has never been accompanied by any indication of paresis. If the story suggests physical weakness, then its distribution, mode of development, manner of recurrence and associated symptoms establish the pattern on which diagnosis of the site of the lesion and of the underlying pathological process rests.

The possible significance of a monoplegic, hemiplegic, paraplegic or quadriplegic distribution of weakness has been outlined. When all four limbs are involved by weakness which is not the result of disturbance of the upper motor neurone, a proximal distribution of weakness suggests that muscle is primarily at fault and a distal distribution favours a lower motor neurone origin, although there are exceptions. The paresis of acute polyradiculitis of the Guillain–Barré type and porphyric polyneuritis may sometimes be more marked in proximal muscles. Dystrophia myotonica and some rare forms of muscular dystrophy may affect distal muscles more severely but these are unlikely to be confused with neurogenic weakness.

A progressive paraparesis or quadriparesis must always arouse the suspicion of spinal cord compression, and a progressive hemiparesis suggests the possibility of cerebral compression.

The pattern of onset of weakness and the presence or absence of any fluctuation in severity, is a guide to the aetiology. The intermittent course of cerebral vascular insufficiency, the stepwise progression of cerebral thrombosis or the more prolonged exacerbations and remissions of multiple sclerosis often point to the diagnosis. The recurrent paralyses of hypokalaemia are another characteristic pattern of weakness, which may be borne out by the family history. Loss of weight, polyuria, vomiting, diarrhoea, cough and other general symptoms alert the clinician to the possibility of carcinoma or metabolic and endocrine disorders as a cause of weakness.

Once a careful history has been obtained, one should have a clear idea of whether weakness is a symptom of a psychological or systemic disorder or of neurological or muscular origin. One can then concentrate on the appropriate points in physical examination.

Examination of the motor system starts with observation of the patient's gait to ensure that the arms swing freely, that balance is maintained without undue separation of the legs; that the legs are not lifted higher than necessary, that neither foot drags, and that turning is executed smoothly. When the patient is lying on the examination couch, the posture of the patient is noted, then the presence of any muscular wasting, fasciculation or involuntary movements. Muscle tone is then assessed by observation of the way in which the limbs are maintained in position against gravity when the patient's eyes are closed and by moving the limbs through their full range of movement several times, increasing the velocity of muscle stretch on each occasion. Power is tested systematically, abductors before adductors and flexors before extensors. A rigid adherence to this routine makes it obvious to the examiner when certain synergies are affected differentially, such as the weakness of flexor groups which characterizes upper motor neurone weakness in the lower limbs. Rapid repetitive and alternating movements may then be examined, followed by co-ordination tests to provide a further assessment of control by upper motor neurone and cerebellum. The deep and superficial reflexes are examined with the patient lying supine in a convenient position to test symmetry. For example, the radial reflexes are first examined with the upper limbs partly flexed at the elbow and the hands lying comfortably on the patient's trunk. The percussion hammer is then flicked lightly from one radial styloid process to the other and the reflex contraction observed, not only in brachioradialis but in biceps and possibly other muscles in the arms and forearm. The mechanism and significance of the tendon jerk is discussed in the next chapter.

If upper motor neurone weakness is bilateral its upper level must be sought as assiduously as one seeks a sensory level. When the lower limbs appear to be affected exclusively, the patient is asked to lift his head from the examination couch and to try to sit up without using the arms. If the umbilicus moves upwards during this attempt, it shows that the lower abdominal muscles are weak and that the motor level lies in the region of the tenth thoracic segment. If both upper and lower abdominal muscles are weak, one observes movement of the chest to see if a level may be detected by involvement of the intercostal muscles. If the upper limbs are involved the level may be determined by the muscle groups affected and changes in the deep reflexes. If the level is higher than the cervical spinal cord one must pay particular attention to the cranial nerves, including jaw and facial jerks. In this way an apparent paraparesis may be shown to be a quadriparesis from a lesion of the cervical spinal cord or its origin may be found in the brain-stem or cerebral hemispheres. A number of different foci of involvement of the motor system may be detected in multiple sclerosis, combined cervical and lumbar spondylosis, neurofibromatosis, meningitis carcinomatosa, metastatic tumours, neurosyphilis and sarcoidosis.

SUMMARY

Weakness may be a subjective sensation, or a loss of muscle power which can be assessed objectively. Asthenia may be confused with myasthenia. Asthenia is a subjective feeling of physical tiredness with a host of organic and psychosomatic causes. Myasthenia is a progressive failure of muscle contraction with objective signs of weakness after exertion.

Paralysis or paresis may result from disturbance of the upper motor neurone (comprising the pyramidal tract and its associated extrapyramidal pathways), or from the lower motor neurone, the neuromuscular junction or muscle. The distribution of weakness, the manner of its evolution and the nature of the accompanying symptoms and physical signs usually indicate the site of the disorder. Various causes of hemiparesis, quadriparesis and paraparesis are mentioned, as well as common disorders which may affect the lower motor neurone, neuromuscular junction or muscle. Hysterical weakness may be distinguished from paresis of organic origin by observing the simultaneous contraction of agonists and antagonists, and the lack of counter-pressure in the opposite limb.

The clinical significance of the history and the importance of systematic examination of the motor system is described as a preliminary to the analysis of motor phenomena in the following chapters.

REFERENCES

[1] Eccles, J. C. (1964). *The Physiology of Synapses.* Pp. 11–13, 29–36, 60, Berlin; Springer

[2] Karczmar, A. G. (1967). 'Neuromuscular pharmacology.' *A. Rev. Pharmac.* **7**, 241–276

[3] Lambert, E. H. and Rooke, E. D. (1965). 'Myasthenic state and lung cancer.' In *The Remote Effects of Cancer on the Nervous System.* Ed. by W. R. Brain and F. H. Norris Jr. New York; Grune and Stratton

[4] McQuillen, M. P. and Johns, R. J. (1963). 'Asthenic syndrome. Anticholinesterase tolerance in non-myasthenic patients.' *Archs Neurol.* **8**, 382–387

[5] Preswick, G. and Henderson, A. S. (1965). 'Myasthenia and the "asthenic" syndrome.' *Med. J. Aust.* **1**, 335–337

[6] Roberts, H. J. (1964). 'Chronic refractory fatigue—an "organic" perspective.' *Med. Times N.Y.* **92**, 1144

[7] Simpson, J. A. (1966). 'Disorders of neuromuscular transmission.' *Proc. R. Soc. Med.* **59**, 993–998

[8] Simpson, J. A. (1962). 'The neuropathies.' In *Modern Trends in Neurology–3*, pp. 245–291. London; Butterworths

[9] Walton, J. N. (Ed.) (1969). *Disorders of Voluntary Muscle.* London; Churchill

3—The Tendon Jerk: A Phasic Stretch Reflex

Eliciting the muscle reflexes or tendon jerks is such an important part of the examination of the nervous system that the percussion hammer could be regarded as a symbol of the neurologist. An understanding of the mechanism of the tendon jerk is essential for an intelligent appraisal of the function of the spinal cord at various segmental levels and of the motor system in general. The analysis of this mechanism is a useful starting-point for a discussion of the motor system, since much of the neuronal superstructure which has evolved for the control of movement exerts its action at the segmental level of the spinal cord. The physiology of the stretch reflex arc is considered first as a prelude to the clinical significance of the tendon jerk in man.

THE STRETCH REFLEX

The stretch reflex should be the simplest of all central reflexes to understand because it consists of only two nerve cells, a receptor and effector neurone. Its apparent simplicity is deceptive for there are many influences which play upon each side of the reflex arc to alter its sensitivity in health and disease.

The stretch reflex has both phasic and tonic components. A tonic stretch reflex is one in which a stimulus produces a prolonged asynchronous discharge of motor neurones causing sustained muscle contraction for the maintenance or alteration of posture. In contrast to this, a phasic stretch reflex consists of a synchronous motor neurone discharge caused by brief stimulation of muscle spindles or their afferent nerve pathways. The tendon jerk is a phasic stretch reflex. The active contraction provoked in a muscle by continuous stretch is a tonic reflex and is the basis of muscle 'tone'. The term

49

muscle tone is used in the clinical sense to mean the active resistance felt from muscle contraction when a joint is passively flexed or extended by the examiner. It does not mean that activity is present in the resting muscle to give the appearance or feeling of firmness to the muscle belly. In the normally relaxed individual the only resistance felt on moving a limb at a joint is that due to the mechanical properties of the limb, its joints, ligaments and muscles. There is no active contraction of muscle to be demonstrated electrically by leads attached to the skin over the surface of the muscle, that is, there is no tonic stretch reflex. If the subject is then asked to clench one hand, or turn the head from side to side, or make some difficult calculation, he or she tenses, stretch reflexes appear and active resistance can be felt on manipulation of a joint.

Some subjects are habitually tense and are quite unable to relax. These people have palpable stretch reflexes, which may be so marked as to give a feeling of rigidity to the limb. If, in addition, they have an exaggerated physiological tremor, as so many anxious people do, the stretch reflex is fragmented by the tremor rhythm to give a 'cogwheel' effect which resembles that of Parkinson's disease. Thus something happens in normal subjects who are alerted by mental concentration, anticipation or physical activity to bring the stretch reflex into operation, to 'switch it on' or render it more sensitive, and the same mechanism appears to operate continuously in tense anxious individuals so that they are unable to 'switch off'.

The historical importance of decerebrate rigidity

It had been known before the time of Sherrington that damage to the forebrain of animals would give rise to stiffness of the limbs, particularly of the extensor muscles, so that the animal would stand if carefully placed upright. Liddell and Sherrington[16] analysed this phenomenon of decerebrate rigidity and found that it depended upon a spinal cord reflex which they termed the stretch reflex. Muscles of the decerebrate animal responded to a given degree of stretch with a much greater contraction than those of a normal animal. The rigidity disappeared immediately the dorsal roots were cut, indicating that nerve impulses maintaining rigidity were passing along afferent fibres from the limb and causing muscle contraction by reflexly discharging motor neurones. Sherrington found that it was necessary to isolate the brain substance from the spinal cord at the mid-brain level, in the vicinity of the red nucleus, to produce the full pattern of decerebrate rigidity. Destruction of the red nucleus alone has since been shown to have no effect on muscle tone, although the neighbouring reticular formation has a powerful action which will be discussed later. Sherrington observed that the decerebrate animal retained its abnormal tone and posture while sections were made caudally down the brain-stem until the vestibular nucleus was reached. As soon as the vestibular nucleus was damaged the rigidity melted away. It therefore appeared that the removal of some cerebral control mechanism whose descending pathway traversed the mid-brain would release the pattern of extensor rigidity, and that withdrawal of vestibulospinal activity would abolish it permanently. The phenomenon was thus caused by the enhancement of the tonic stretch reflex in extensor muscles as a result of imbalance of the supraspinal influences which normally regulate the reflex. Sherrington also discovered that stimulation of a cutaneous nerve in a decerebrate animal inhibited the stretch reflex in extensor muscles of the same limb and induced flexion of the limb, thus establishing the principle of reciprocal innervation between antagonists.

Since that time, our knowledge of the stretch reflex has grown in detail but has not altered in principle. The reflex arc is known to depend upon an afferent fibre arising from receptors within the specialized muscle fibres of the muscle spindle which synapses with a motor neurone, whose axon supplies muscle fibres surrounding the spindle (*Figure 3.1*).

THE MUSCLE SPINDLE

The anatomy of the muscle spindle is now well established, although there is still some dispute about the fine details of its innervation. Each muscle spindle is less than a centimetre long and consists of 2–12 intrafusal fibres (usually about 10 in man) in an envelope of connective tissue, lying in parallel with the surrounding muscle fibres. Spindles are distributed throughout flexor and extensor muscles, more densely in small muscles serving fine movement. In most muscles, the spindles are distributed throughout the belly of the muscle with their greatest concentration near the main intra-muscular nerves.

On histological examination, two types of fibre may be recognized within the spindle capsule. One has contractile muscular ends and a central dilatation containing nuclei, while the other is a ribbon or chain-like fibre containing nuclei throughout its length. Both 'nuclear-bag' and 'nuclear-chain' fibres have a receptor in their central regions, known as a primary ending, which is usually annulospiral in appearance (*Figure 3.1*). Some nuclear-bag fibres and all nuclear-chain fibres contain additional secondary endings which are diffusely applied throughout the length of the fibre apart from the central region and are termed 'flower-spray' endings because of their appearance. Both types of spindle fibres (intrafusal fibres) are supplied by small motor (gamma efferent) nerves, which enable the striated polar regions of the intrafusal fibre to contract. The terms alpha and gamma efferent are used to describe the motor supply to extrafusal and intrafusal fibres respectively because their calibre is comparable with the alpha and gamma groups described by Erlanger and Gasser[8] when they classified the action potentials

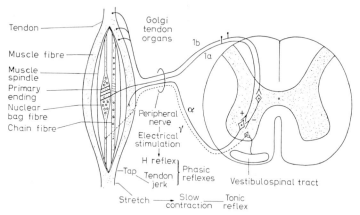

Figure 3.1. The monosynaptic reflex crc. Group Ia afferent fibres from nuclear bag and nuclear chain fibres of the muscle spindle synapse directly upon the large alpha motor neurones in the anterior horn, whose axons cause the muscle fibres surrounding the spindle to contract. The alpha cell is inhibited through an interneurone by group Ib afferent fibres from Golgi tendon organs. The gamma efferent system supplying the contractile ends of muscle spindle fibres is regulated by descending motor pathways, one of which, the vestibulospinal tract, is illustrated. Secondary spindle endings and group II afferent fibres are not shown

of peripheral nerves according to conduction velocity. Some efferent fibres of intermediate velocity (beta fibres) supply both muscle and spindle fibres[1]. The gamma efferent system is being studied further because of variation in the calibre of its axons and the nature of its endings on spindle fibres (endplate and trail endings) which may be correlated with static and dynamic qualities of spindle response[1]. Any subdivision of the gamma system has no clinical significance at the moment.

Both primary and secondary sensory endorgans in spindle fibres respond to the static stimulus of sustained stretch, but primary endings have the additional dynamic quality of being readily stimulated by the velocity of a brief stretch and also by vibration, which presumably imparts a series of brief stretches to the nuclear bag because of its sinusoidal wave-form. Static and dynamic properties of muscle spindles make them suitable as receptors for both tonic and phasic reflexes[20].

Since the muscle spindles lie among ordinary striated fibres and are in parallel with them, they are relieved by tension when the surrounding muscle contracts, so that they discharge impulses more slowly or cease to fire altogether. If spindle fibres were unable to contract themselves so that their discharge ceased with every muscle contraction, reflex muscle contraction would undergo a regular sequence of on–off reactions. A stretch would induce a reflex muscle contraction which unloaded the spindle, thereby stopping its discharge of impulses and causing the reflex contraction of muscle to cease, thus restoring the load on the spindle once more. Under normal circumstances, however, the potential for such fluctuations in stretch reflex activity is reduced by the intrafusal fibres themselves contracting, since they are innervated by the small motor nerves of the gamma efferent system[14]. The effect of gamma efferent activity is to sensitize the spindle endings to a stretch stimulus because the non-contractile central portion of the nuclear bag fibre elongates when its polar regions contract and its contained receptors are deformed. The primary ending is thus given an initial base-line stretch or 'bias' by virtue of contraction of the intrafusal fibres so that it will respond more readily to any externally applied stimulus, such as direct stretch or a vibration wave. The gamma efferent system may therefore be regarded as a control of the sensitivity of the stretch reflex arc, which may be adjusted up or down by central influences.

It can be seen that the signal transmitted from spindle endings varies as the ratio of spindle contraction to that of its surrounding muscle fibres. If the spindle is contracted relatively more than surrounding muscle, its firing rate is increased and its reflex effects tend to cause contraction of the surrounding muscle, thus reaching the resting state at a shorter length. If the spindle is slack relative to surrounding muscle, its firing rate decreases, and its diminished reflex effects tend to produce relaxation of surrounding muscle, thus restoring the resting state at a greater muscle length. It can therefore be said that spindle receptors act as detectors of discrepancies or error between length of spindles and that of surrounding muscle fibres, and that the gamma efferent activity or bias helps to determine the final length of the muscle fibres surrounding the spindle[22].

53

When the muscle tendon is tapped, the gamma bias determines the force of the signal generated by the muscle spindle and hence the degree to which a phasic reflex contraction will occur assuming the sensitivity of the alpha motor neurones remains constant. When the muscle is stretched, the gamma and alpha bias determine the force of tonic muscle contraction with which the stretch is reflexly resisted.

Afferent fibres from muscle

Apart from the muscle spindle, there are other receptors associated with muscle such as Golgi tendon organs, free nerve endings and Pacinian corpuscles. Golgi tendon organs are not only in tendons but are scattered throughout muscle bellies at musculotendinous junctions. They are in series with muscle fibres and respond to tension whether it is applied by stretching the muscle through manipulation of the appropriate joint, or by active contraction of the muscle itself. Golgi tendon organs require a greater degree of passive stretch than the muscle spindle for the initiation of impulses but respond readily to active contraction of muscle fibres because of their site at the point of attachment of muscle fibres. The central effect of their discharge is to inhibit the stretch reflex through an interneurone (*Figure 3.1*).

Pacinian corpuscles are probably responsible for conscious perception of vibration and deep pressure from muscle, and the free nerve endings for painful sensation.

The afferent fibres which carry impulses from primary spindle endings and also those from Golgi tendon organs are of wide diameter, conduct rapidly, and are known as Ia and Ib fibres respecttively. The afferents from secondary spindle endings are of smaller calibre, slower conduction velocity and are termed group II. Group I and II afferents pass centrally in the muscle nerve then join cutaneous afferents to form a mixed peripheral nerve. They pass into the spinal cord through the posterior root, their cell bodies being contained in the root ganglion, to enter the posterior horn of grey matter (*Figure 3.1*). Group Ia fibres then sweep directly to the anterior horn of grey matter on the same side of the spinal cord where they synapse with motor neurones (alpha cells) whose large diameter axons pass out in the anterior root and down peripheral nerve to complete the monosynaptic stretch reflex arc. Group Ib fibres suppress the activity of motor neurones by means of an intermediate inhibitory neurone. Group II fibres, which are not illustrated in *Figure 3.1*, have differential central effects through interneurones, tending to facilitate flexor motor neurones and to inhibit extensor motor neurones.

The axons of motor neurones branch while still within the spinal cord and these recurrent collaterals synapse with a small cell, the Renshaw cell. The Renshaw cell inhibits anterior horn cell activity for a period of up to 100 milliseconds, thus preventing repetitive firing of the anterior horn cell in response to a single stimulus.

PHASIC MUSCLE REFLEXES

The term phasic when applied here to stretch reflexes means that the afferent and efferent discharge is relatively synchronous. The term may also be applied to transient movements to distinguish them from slow muscle contraction maintaining posture. Phasic is used in this sense later in the discussion of movement.

The H reflex

It is possible to stimulate muscle afferent fibres electrically wherever the peripheral nerve containing them lies close to the surface. Group I muscle afferent fibres are of larger diameter than efferent fibres and have a conduction velocity some 10 per cent greater[6, 19]. They are of lower threshold and probably lie superficial to efferent fibres in the medial popliteal nerve. For these reasons, they may usually be stimulated selectively as shown in *Figure 3.2*. A synchronous nerve impulse is thus initiated in group I fibres, which traverses the monosynaptic stretch reflex arc to produce a sharp reflex contraction in the calf muscles resembling the response to tendon tap[18]. This is termed the H reflex after P. Hoffmann who first described it in 1918. The H reflex arc is essentially the same as that of the ankle jerk except that the muscle spindle receptors are by-passed by stimulating the afferent nerve directly[17]. Both tendon jerk and H reflexes are phasic reflexes being of brief duration, relying on synchronous afferent and reflex efferent volleys. The H reflex has been studied extensively[21] and provides a useful method for investigating alpha motor neurone excitability free from direct influence of the gamma efferent system. There is an indirect influence in that discharge from muscle spindles provides a background of facilitation for the H reflex, which is shown by the depression of the H reflex when spindle sensitivity is impaired by blockade of the gamma efferent system with intrathecal procaine[2].

Reinforcement of tendon jerks by clenching the hands or pulling one hand against the other (Jendrassik manoeuvre) operates mainly by increasing the activity in the gamma efferent system but must also have an effect on alpha cells, since some increase in amplitude of H reflexes occurs during reinforcement, even after gamma efferent block which rules out an indirect effect via the gamma loop and spindle afferents[12,13]. The H reflex is subject to periodic fluctuations in amplitude, because of central influences affecting alpha and gamma cells which change according to the state of alertness of the subject[3,23].

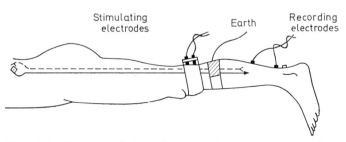

Figure 3.2. Placement of electrodes to record the monosynaptic reflex in man, induced by electrical stimulation of group Ia fibres in the medial popliteal nerve (H reflex)

To obtain the H reflex alone, the intensity of stimulation has to be carefully controlled, as a slight increase will excite efferent as well as afferent fibres and a direct muscle response (M response) then appears with a short latency (*Figure 3.3*). When a nerve fibre is adequately stimulated, the resulting discharge spreads not only in the direction in which the nerve normally conducts (orthodromic volley) but also in the reverse direction (antidromic volley). In the case of the medial popliteal and sciatic nerves, the afferent volley discharges the anterior horn cell and the post-synaptic volley is on its way down motor fibres when it meets the antidromic impulses travelling in the opposite direction. The two volleys collide and the propagation of the H reflex is prevented. This can be demonstrated by increasing the intensity of stimulation of the medial popliteal nerve. The direct muscle response becomes larger and the H reflex progressively smaller (*Figures 3.3, 3.4*). To minimize excitation of motor fibres, the stimulus voltage is usually restricted to 1·1 or 1·2 threshold, that is, the voltage required to produce the smallest discernible H reflex.

The H reflex has qualities similar to the monosynaptic stretch reflex of animals. Repetitive stimulation of the monosynaptic arc in the cat will cause an increase in excitability of the reflex lasting for some minutes after stimulation ceases, probably because of increased mobilization of transmitter substance at the synapse[5,7,15]. This phenomenon, known as post-tetanic potentiation, has also been demonstrated for the H reflex in man [4,9]. During the period of post-tetanic potentiation of the H reflex, contraction of the antagonistic muscles (the ankle dorsiflexors) is partially inhibited, illustrating the presence of reciprocal innervation

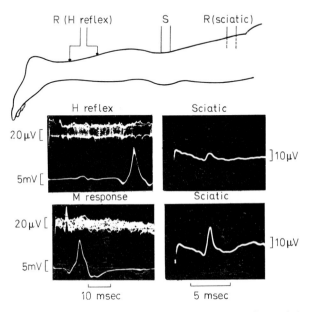

Figure 3.3. Comparison of the sciatic nerve potential recorded in man by depth electrodes with soleus muscle potential when the medial popliteal nerve is stimulated as in Figure 3.2, at different intensities. The stimulus can be adjusted to produce an almost pure afferent volley and H reflex, as seen in the upper panels. When the intensity is increased so that efferent fibres are also stimulated, the H reflex volley is occluded in the motor limb of the reflex arc by the antidromic efferent volley. The direct muscle response (M response) is then predominant (lower panels)

Post-tetanic potentiation of phasic reflexes is rather variable in man and requires further study to assess the circumstances which produce it, and the variability of its degree and time course in normal subjects, before it can be applied to the investigation of neurological disorder.

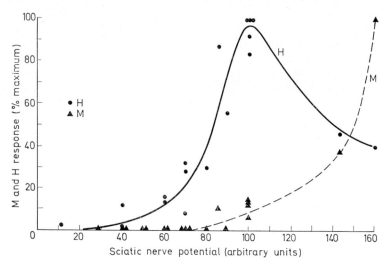

Figure 3.4. Correlation of sciatic nerve potential with H reflex and M response in man, showing the decline of the H reflex as more efferent fibres become active when stimulus intensity is progressively increased

The tendon jerk

Both tendon jerk and H reflex are produced by a stimulus which is so brief as to be unnatural. There must be few occasions in life when a sudden undirected reflex contraction of limb muscles in response to a sharp blow could serve any useful purpose. Whether or not the jerk itself has any physiological significance it is a means of testing the integrity of the stretch reflex arc and the activity of alpha (and indirectly, gamma) motor neurones at any level. The anterior horn cells are responsible for maintaining tonic contraction of muscle and for mediating voluntary movement, so that assessment of their activity assumes great importance as a clinical test. Since muscles are innervated by different segmental levels throughout the neuraxis, the tendon jerk provides a means of sampling motor cell excitability at many brain-stem and spinal cord levels (Table 3.1). Phasic muscle reflexes ('tendon jerks') are elicited by a sharp blow to the body in the vicinity of the muscle to be tested, which is most effective if given to the tendon of a partly stretched muscle, but can also be effective when applied to the muscle belly or to bone if the reflex arc is sufficiently excitable. The most suitable blow is a flicking movement which retracts the percussion hammer rapidly so that vibration waves set up in the limb by percussion are not damped down. The nature of the effective stimulus is a brief stretch applied to the muscle spindle which initiates an afferent volley in group Ia nerves fibres. The stretch may be applied directly, but, in many postures, it is probable that a vibration wave travelling through the

TABLE 3.1

Levels of the Central Nervous System at which Segmental Mechanisms may be Tested by Reflex Activity

Level		Deep (muscle) reflex	Other reflexes
Cranial	2, 3		Pupillary light response
Cranial	5	Jaw	
	7	Facial	
	5, 7		Corneal
	9, 10, 11		Gag
Spinal	C5, 6	Biceps	
		Brachioradialis (radial)	
	7	Triceps	
	8	Finger	
	T7–9	Abdominal, upper	Abdominal upper
	10–12	,, lower	,, lower
	L1		Cremasteric
	L3–4	Quadriceps (knee jerk)	
	L5, S1–2	Hamstrings	
	S1	Gastrocnemius-soleus (ankle jerk)	
			Plantar
	S2, 3		Bulbo-cavernosus
	S3, 4, 5		Anal

muscle belly is responsible for stimulating the spindle by inducing a rapid sinusoidal oscillation of the spindle (*Figure 3.5*). This can be seen most clearly in subjects with brisk reflexes in whom a blow which is clearly in the wrong direction to produce a direct stretch of the muscle fibre will nevertheless induce a strong reflex contraction (Figure 3.6).

In many normal subjects, percussion of the radius will provoke reflex contraction not only of the brachioradialis but of biceps and finger flexors as well. Close observation will often disclose that finger extensors, triceps and pectoralis major contract at the same time. This phenomenon, known as reflex irradiation or 'spread', is particularly noticeable in patients with spasticity in whom reflex contraction may be seen in most muscles of the same side and also some on the side opposite to the blow given. In the lower limbs, contraction of the hamstrings muscles and thigh adductors often accompanies elicitation of the ankle jerk by percussion of the tendo achillis. The quadriceps may also contract reflexly and adductors of the opposite limb may contract (crossed adductor jerk). All

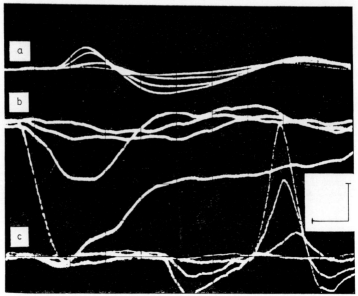

Figure 3.5. Knee jerk increasing in proportion to vibration evoked by tapping ligamentum patellae. The amplitude of the quadriceps muscle potential (c) increases proportionately to the vibration wave recorded over the muscle belly (a), and not to velocity of muscle stretch as gauged by a displacement transducer impinging on the patella (b). Calibration: vertical, 0·2mV; horizontal, 5 ms.

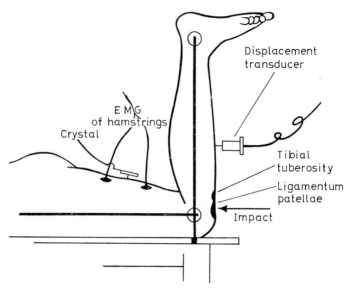

Figure 3.6. Hamstrings jerk induced by vibration. Diagram of experimental arrangement to demonstrate hamstrings jerk elicited by a blow to the ligamentum patellae when the limb is braced so that the hamstring muscles are not stretched

these 'irradiated' or 'indirect' reflexes can be accounted for satisfactorily in terms of their nature and latency by the propagation of a vibration wave from the point of percussion of the limb[10,11]. The vibration wave passes from bone to muscle, stimulating any susceptible muscle spindle which lies in its path. The possibility of any

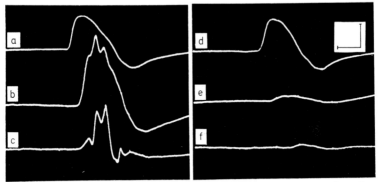

Figure 3.7. Persistence of biceps contraction in response to tapping radius after ischaemic block of forearm. (a), (b), (c), show reflex contractions of biceps, brachioradialis and finger flexors following radial tap. (d), (e), (f), as above, after 30 minutes' ischaemia of forearm. Brachioradialis and finger jerks have disappeared, without any change in amplitude of biceps potential, showing that the proximal irradiation of reflexes does not depend upon nerve impulses from the periphery (Reproduced from Lance and de Gail[11] by courtesy of the Editor of J. Neurol. Neurosurg. Psychiat.)

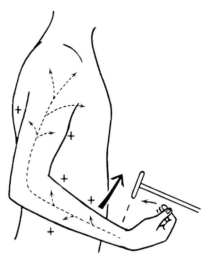

Figure 3.8. Muscle contractions produced by radial tap in a subject with brisk reflexes. The propagation of a vibration wave through the limb initiates reflex contractions (+) in biceps, triceps, brachioradialis, finger flexors and extensors. The limb moves in the direction of the stronger muscles so that the elbow and fingers flex, the reaction of a normal 'supinator' or radial jerk

neural pathways being responsible for the reflex contraction of muscles remote from the point percussed has been eliminated by experiments using ischaemic block of peripheral nerve fibres (*Figure 3.7*). The concept of vibration being the means of applying the brief stretch essential for the tendon jerk and for irradiation of muscle reflexes is illustrated in *Figure 3.8*. The importance of vibration in the elicitation of muscle reflexes was foreshadowed by Wartenberg[24,25] in a critical study of reflexes in clinical use when he pointed out that jarring of muscle was the essential stimulus and that concussion of bone transmitted the 'mechanical insult' to the muscle concerned. It is well worth reading Wartenberg's review to see the profusion of reflexes which are based on this principle and which have been endowed with the name of some clinician who achieved an ephemeral memorial by tapping a different bony prominence.

THE CLINICAL SIGNIFICANCE OF THE TENDON JERK

The understanding of the mechanism of deep muscle reflexes explains a number of common clinical phenomena which appear when some reflex pathways are active while others are blocked. If, for example, there is a lesion of the fifth and sixth cervical segments which mediate the biceps and brachioradialis reflexes, these muscles are unable to respond to a vibration wave by reflex contraction. Provided that there is suitable gamma efferent activity in other muscles of the limb, the other muscles will continue to respond reflexly to a vibration wave. In these circumstances, percussion of the radius which usually causes a flexion movement of the upper limb (radial, supinator or brachioradialis jerk) will induce contraction of those muscles whose reflex arc remains intact, that is, of the finger flexors and triceps. The upper limb thus extends at the elbow and the fingers flex, a response which has been called the 'inverted supinator jerk' (*Figure 3.9*). There is obviously nothing paradoxical or 'inverted' about such a response. Movements of finger flexors and triceps are frequently provoked by radial tap but are not often observed because of the more obvious contraction in biceps and brachioradialis. They are simply revealed by blockade of the C5–6 reflex pathways. If the lesion involving these segments is compressing the spinal cord as well as the C5–6 nerve roots, gamma efferent discharge may well be increased below this segmental level so that triceps and finger jerks are exaggerated, thus accentuating the phenomenon. Extension of the wrist may occasionally be seen in response to radial tap if there is a lesion of the eighth cervical segment which diminishes the usually dominant response in the flexors. In routine clinical examination when the biceps muscle or finger flexors are seen to contract in response to percussion of the radius, it is unnecessary to tap the biceps tendon separately or to elicit the finger jerks directly, since the reflex arc of the biceps and finger flexors has already been tested and proven to be intact by the vibration set up by percussion.

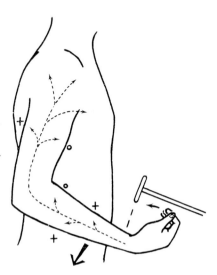

Figure 3.9. The mechanism of 'the inverted supinator jerk'. When reflex arcs employing the fifth and sixth cervical segments are interrupted by disease, the biceps and brachioradialis response to the vibration wave set up by radial tap is absent (o). Reflex contraction of triceps, finger flexors and extensors, whose reflex arcs are intact respond normally (+). The elbow thus extends while fingers flex

If the thumb flexes when the finger jerks are elicited by tapping the fingers, this indicates that the muscle spindles of thumb flexors are in a suitable state of gamma bias to respond to the propagated vibration wave. This is almost certainly the mechanism of 'Hoffmann's sign', a reflex flexion of the thumb in response to snapping the terminal phalanx of the index or middle finger. Hoffmann's sign does not necessarily indicate an upper motor neurone lesion since many normal subjects have sufficient gamma bias to show this response.

When gamma bias is adequate, a brief twitch of abdominal muscles may be obtained by percussion over the rib cage or pelvis. This contraction is mediated through the same thoracic segments which normally serve the superficial abdominal reflexes, but is dependent upon muscle receptors responding to stretch or vibration, and not skin receptors responding to touch. In the lower limb, percussion of the tendo achillis or the malleoli may evoke contraction of hamstrings, thigh adductors and sometimes (depending upon limb position and the degree of alpha and gamma bias) the quadriceps, thus effectively testing the reflex arcs of each of these muscles.

Clinical examination of muscle reflexes therefore consists of supplying an input to varying levels of the nervous system and estimating the output. If the level of gamma bias to muscle spindles or alpha motor neurone excitability is generally low, tendon jerks will be diminished or absent. In this case 'reinforcement' of the reflexes by requesting the subject to contract some muscle elsewhere in the body or to contract gently the muscle whose reflex is being elicited, or by increasing the mental alertness of the subject, will increase alpha and gamma efferent activity, and hence the muscle spindle response and the tendon jerk. If alpha and gamma bias is high, which is common in tense apprehensive subjects, as well as patients with upper motor neurone lesions, the tendon jerks will be brisk. If alpha and gamma bias is extreme, relaxation of the muscle after the reflex twitch has finished will load muscle spindles sufficiently to make them fire again, so that a succession of muscle twitches is observed because of repetitive firing of the stretch reflex arc. If gentle stretch is applied to the muscle, for example, steady pressure dorsiflexing the foot in the case of the ankle jerk, the reflex arc will be discharged rhythmically at the rate of 6–7 muscle twitches each second, a phenomenon known as clonus. The fact that a few beats of clonus may be seen in nervous but normal individuals is not surprising, since alpha and gamma bias may be functionally enhanced in anxious people. In most instances, sustained clonus is a sign of an upper motor neurone lesion.

It is important to look for discrepancy or asymmetry of phasic stretch reflexes on examination of a patient, since little importance can be attached to a generalized diminution or generalized enhancement of the reflexes, unless this is associated with convincing associated signs of a diffuse lower motor neurone lesion, such as polyneuritis, or a bilateral upper motor neurone disturbance such as spastic quadriparesis. The general level of reflex activity must therefore be determined for a particular subject and its departure from normal, if any, assessed. Attention may then be given to any asymmetry which may indicate a segmental or peripheral nerve lesion by depression of the response, or an upper motor neurone lesion by its relative briskness. Depression of reflexes in distal muscles relative to proximal muscles may also be of significance in indicating a peripheral neuritis or bilateral compression of the appropriate nerve roots, but it must be borne in mind that distal reflexes are often diminished in the elderly as a part of the normal ageing process. Examination of the deep muscle reflexes is thus an essential part of the neurological examination, but must be interpreted in physiological terms as a part of the whole clinical picture.

SUMMARY

Muscle contracts reflexly in response to stretch. A tonic contraction is produced by slow stretch in a suitably tense individual, and a phasic contraction is produced by a sharp stretch or sudden vibration applied to muscle. The receptors for the stretch reflex are contained in muscle spindles, lying in parallel with ordinary muscle fibres. Group Ia afferent fibres from the muscle spindle synapse with alpha motor neurones in the anterior horn of the spinal cord, which form the efferent limb of the reflex, causing the muscle fibres surrounding the spindle to contract in response to stretch. The excitability of spindle afferents is governed by the degree of tension in the centre of the spindle fibre which is determined by the contraction induced in the spindle by its own motor supply, the small-fibred gamma efferent system. The gamma efferent system is governed by supraspinal pathways and is not a part of the stretch reflex arc although it is one of the factors which determines its sensitivity. Gamma efferent activity or bias helps to control the length of voluntary muscle by the stretch reflex arc and may be responsible for the initiation of some movements.

A brisk tap on muscle tendon or a blow to the limb sets up a vibration wave which propagates from bone to muscle, thus inducing a brief stretch of the spindle and causing a muscle contraction mediated by the stretch reflex arc. A similar reflex contraction, obtained by electrical stimulation of the muscle nerve, by-passing the spindle mechanism, is termed the H reflex. Both tendon jerk and H reflex may be enhanced by processes of reinforcement which increase the excitability of both alpha and gamma cells.

The tendon jerk affords a useful method of testing the integrity of the reflex arc at various spinal segmental levels in man, and of assessing the activity of both alpha and gamma motor systems at these levels. Clinical phenomena such as the irradiation of reflexes and the inverted supinator jerk are explained in terms of vibration being the means by which percussion applies a brief stretch to the muscles concerned.

REFERENCES

[1] Barker, D. (1967). 'The innervation of mammalian skeletal muscle. In *Myotatic, Kinesthetic and Vestibular Mechanisms*. Ciba Foundation Symposium pp. 3–19. Ed. by A. V. S. de Reuck and K. Knight; London; Churchill

[2] Clare, M. H. and Landau, W. M. (1964). 'Fusimotor function—Part V. Reflex reinforcement under fusimotor block in normal subjects.' *Archs. Neurol.* **10**, 123–127

[3] Coquery, J-M. (1962). *Les variations 'spontanées' du reflexe de Hoffmann.* Thesis, Université d'Aix-Marseille

[4] Corrie, W. S. and Hardin, W. B. (1964). 'Post-tetanic potentiation of H reflex in normal man.' *Archs Neurol.* **11**, 317–323

[5] Curtis, D. and Eccles, J. C. (1962). 'Synaptic action during and after repetitive stimulation.' *J. Physiol. Lond.* **150**, 374–398

[6] Diamantopoulos, E. and Gassel, M. M. (1965). 'Electrically induced monosynaptic reflexes in man.' *J. Neurol. Neurosurg. Psychiat.* **28**, 496–502

[7] Eccles, J. C. and Rall, W. (1951). 'Effects induced in a monosynaptic reflex path by its activation.' *J. Neurophysiol.* **14**, 353–376

[8] Erlanger, J. and Gasser, H. S. (1937). *Electrical Signs of Nervous Activity.* Philadelphia; Univ. of Pennsylvania Press

[9] Hagbarth, K-E. (1962). 'Post-tetanic potentiation of myotatic reflexes in man.' *J. Neurol. Neurosurg. Psychiat.* **25**, 1–10

[10] Lance, J. W. (1965). 'The mechanism of reflex irradiation.' *Proc. Aust. Ass. Neurol.* **3**, 77–81

[11] Lance, J. W. and de Gail, P. (1965). 'Spread of phasic muscle reflexes in normal and spastic subjects.' *J. Neurol. Neurosurg. Psychiat.* **28**, 328–334

[12] Lance, J. W., Schwab, R. S. and Peterson, E. A. (1963). 'Action tremor and the cogwheel phenomenon in Parkinson's disease.' *Brain* **86**, 95–110

[13] Landau, W. M. and Clare, M. H. (1964). 'Fusimotor function, part IV. Reinforcement of the H reflex in normal subjects.' *Archs Neurol.* **10**, 117–122

[14] Leksell, L. (1945). 'The action potential and excitatory effects of the small ventral root fibres to skeletal muscle.' *Acta physiol. scand.* Suppl. **31**, 1–84

[15] Lloyd, D. P. C. (1949). 'Post-tetanic potentiation of response in monosynaptic reflex pathways of the spinal cord.' *J. gen. Physiol.* **33**, 147–170

[16] Liddell, E. G. T. and Sherrington, C. S. (1924). 'Reflexes in response to stretch (myotatic reflexes).' *Proc. R. Soc.* **96B**, 212–242

[17] Magladery, J. W. (1955). 'Some observations on spinal reflexes in man.' *Pflügers Arch. ges. Physiol.* **261**, 302–321

[18] Magladery, J. W. and McDougal, D. B. Jr. (1950). 'Electro-physiological studies of nerve and reflex activity in normal man. 1. Identification of certain reflexes in the electromyogram and the conduction velocity of peripheral nerve fibres.' *Bull. Johns Hopkins Hosp.* **86**, 265–290

[19] Magladery, J. W., Porter, W. E., Park, A. M. and Teasdall, R. D. (1951). 'Electrophysiological studies of nerve and reflex activity in normal man IV. The two-neurone reflex and identification of certain action potentials from spinal roots and cord.' *Bull. Johns Hopkins Hosp.* **88**, 499–519

[20] Matthews, P. B. C. (1964). 'Muscle spindles and their motor control.' *Physiol. Rev.* **44**, 219–288

[21] Mayer, R. F. and Mawdsley, C. (1965). 'Studies in man and cat of the significance of the H wave.' *J. Neurol. Neurosurg. Psychiat.* **28**, 201–211

[22] Merton, P. A. (1953). 'Speculations on the servo-control of movement.' In *The Spinal Cord*, pp. 247–260. Ciba Foundation Symposium. Ed. by Wolstenholme. London; Churchill

[23] Paillard, J. (1959). 'Functional organization of afferent innervation of muscle studied in man by monosynaptic testing.' *Am. J. phys. Med.* **38**, 239–247

[24] Wartenberg, R. (1944). 'Studies in reflexes. History, physiology, synthesis and nomenclature: Study I.' *Archs Neurol. Psychiat.*, *Chicago* **51**, 113–133

[25] Wartenberg, R. (1945). 'Studies in reflexes. History physiology, synthesis and nomenclature: Study II.' *Archs Neurol. Psychiat.*, *Chicago* **52**, 341–382

4—Tonic Stretch Reflexes: The Mechanism of Muscle Tone and Movement

The reflex contraction exerted by a muscle when it is stretched is known by the clinician as muscle 'tone'. The term is not really accurate but since it is as firmly entrenched as the equally inadequate term 'tendon jerk' it will be used here. Muscle tone is estimated by observing the posture of the limbs in a relaxed state, and when the limbs are held up against gravity, as well as by observing the nature of spontaneous active movement and sensing the resistance of muscles when the limbs are moved passively.

The posture of a bedridden or partially paralysed patient may be determined by persistently overactive tonic reflexes in flexor or extensor groups of muscles, so that the limbs adopt a certain attitude and finally become fixed in that attitude. The posture of many patients who fail to recover from hemiplegia or have a degenerative condition of the basal ganglia is frequently one of flexion of the upper limbs and extension of the lower limbs (*Figure 4.1*). This is the posture of 'exaggerated reflex standing' for man as the flexors of the upper limbs and extensors of the lower limbs are antigravity muscles in man in the standing position.

When a patient rests his elbows on a table and holds his forearms vertically, muscle tone may be gauged from the angle which the hands make with the forearm in the relaxed position. If muscle tone is diminished on one side, the weight of the hand will cause it to hang lower than the normal side as the wrist and finger extensors are not contracting so forcibly in response to the pull of gravity (*Figure 4.2*). Similarly, the foot will be seen to droop toward the floor when the leg is suspended.

Observation of the gait may show that one arm does not swing as much as the other. In states of hypertonia, spasticity or rigidity, the affected arm has a smaller excursion because of the increased response to stretch of the shoulder muscles (*Figure 4.3*). Conversely, in hypotonic states the affected limb may be seen to swing outwards,

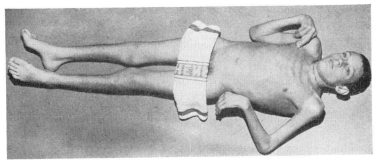

Figure 4.1. Dystonic posture in man, with flexion of upper limbs and extension of lower limbs

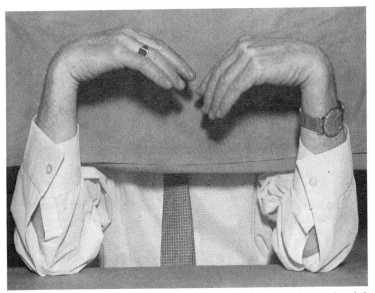

Figure 4.2. Hypotonic posture of the left upper limb in a patient with a left cerebellar lesion. The angle between hand and forearm is less on the left than the right

particularly on turning quickly. The examiner may bring these points out by forcibly and rapidly rotating the shoulders of a standing patient while watching arm movement closely.

Finally, the tonic stretch reflexes for each muscle group may be determined by moving the limbs through their full range of movement at each joint, and estimating whether the force required is more or less than usual. It is necessary to repeat this manoeuvre at different speeds since there may be a certain velocity of stretch which is critical to produce the reflex. In this case, tone may appear to be normal with slow movements, but as the speed is increased, a sudden increase in active resistance or 'catch' will become apparent as the limb is moved.

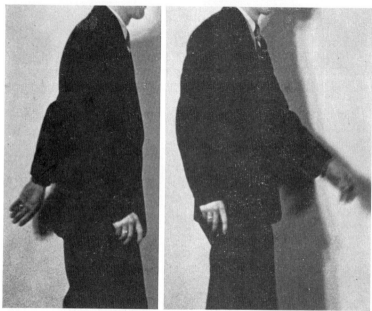

Figure 4.3. Failure to swing one arm when walking. Two frames from a cine-film of a patient with unilateral Parkinson's disease, showing that the rigid right arm moves little while the left arm swings freely

Changes in tonic stretch reflexes do not always run parallel with phasic stretch reflexes, so that one may be faced with the problem of a patient with Parkinson's disease who has increased tone on manipulation of a limb but whose tendon jerks are normal or even diminished. The converse situation of brisk tendon jerks combined with marked hypotonia is commonly seen with cerebellar lesions.

To try to elucidate the reason for the common but puzzling discrepancy between tonic and phasic reflexes in disease, the control of the stretch reflex arc by spinal and supraspinal mechanisms will now be considered.

SPINAL CORD INFLUENCES ON TONIC AND PHASIC REFLEXES

It has long been known that the spinal cord contains inhibitory mechanisms which exert a restraining influence upon extensor muscles. When the spinal cord of a decerebrate cat is severed, extensor tone increases in segments rostral to the level of section (Schiff–Sherrington phenomenon). For example, the forelimbs go into a state of rigidity if the thoracic cord is cut or the quadriceps shows increased stretch reflexes if the lower lumbar cord is transected.

Asphyxia of the spinal cord for about 50 minutes causes destruction of 80 per cent of interneurones with the preservation of large and small motor neurones[12]. The clinical state of animals after this degree of spinal asphyxia is one of extensor rigidity. More extensive asphyxia causes destruction of motor neurones and a flaccid paralysis. Post-ischaemic rigidity has the characteristics of a spastic paraparesis with increased stretch reflexes. It is not abolished by section of the upper cervical cord, indicating that the rigidity is not simply the result of destruction of the terminals of descending inhibitory pathways from the brain-stem. After ischaemia, the monosynaptic arc is normally active but is not inhibited by stimulation of cutaneous nerves, a procedure which usually suppresses extensor reflexes as may be seen when a leg is flexed to avoid a painful stimulus to the sole. Post-tetanic potentiation of the monosynaptic reflex is prolonged after ischaemic damage and extensor neurones fire tonically in response to stretch. In contrast to the activity of the monosynaptic reflex, polysynaptic reflexes are diminished, delayed or absent because of damage to the interneurones on which they depend[32].

These experiments demonstrate clearly that removal of a substantial proportion of spinal cord internuncial cells will cause excessive alpha and gamma motor neurone activity, that is, that there is normally a regulatory effect of spinal interneurones which is responsible, among other activities, for restraining extensor mechanisms.

The limbs can become rigid in man as the result of spinal trauma or of a tumour which infiltrates the spinal cord in such a manner as to isolate the anterior horn cells from internuncial control[39]. Such rigidity may be of the 'alpha' type, that is to say, the resistance to stretch is little altered by procaine block of the gamma efferent system, whereas the alpha cells are hyperactive, both spontaneously and when subject to a normal afferent discharge from stretched muscle. It seems as though the spinal cord possesses networks or 'pools' of neurones capable of facilitating or inhibiting tonic contraction in flexor or extensor muscles, whose activity is not normally apparent but is revealed by disease processes or experimental lesions.

After a single H reflex is discharged through the monosynaptic arc, it takes 5 seconds or more for excitability of the anterior horn cell to return to normal[35]. A similar period of depressed activity follows stimulation of group Ia afferent fibres by a low frequency tetanus or vibration[6]. In patients who have evidence of a lesion a few segments rostral to the level being tested, the phase of late depression after a single H reflex vanishes and the motor neurone becomes normally excitable after a quarter of a second (250 ms)[26]. This suggests that propriospinal fibres normally mediate an inhibitory influence on the anterior horn cell following its discharge singly or repetitively, although at high frequencies of stimulation the local phenomenon of post-tetanic potentiation may overcome such inhibitory influences. The concept of inhibitory and facilitatory pools of intersegmental internuncial neurones which are normally under supraspinal control, is illustrated in *Figure 4.6* (page 76).

Under normal circumstances, spinal influences on tonic and phasic mechanisms are linked, and reciprocal innervation ensures that extensors relax when flexors contract and so on. There are also linkages across the cord so that flexion of one limb is associated with extension of the opposite limb, the crossed extensor response. Reflexes using cervical segments are integrated with lumbar reflexes by propriospinal fibres which may produce a co-ordinated pattern such as walking in four legged animals.

It can be seen that the isolated spinal cord has considerable potential for potentiating or suppressing tonic and phasic mechanisms, and for ensuring that they are normally used in a manner appropriate for purposive action. Further control is imposed upon these mechanisms from higher levels of the nervous system.

SUPRASPINAL CONTROL OF MOTOR NEURONES

Spinal patterns of posture and movement are normally subject to control by pyramidal and extrapyramidal pathways. Some measure of influence is brought to bear by postural reflexes mediated through the brain-stem, such as the tonic neck reflexes and tonic labyrinthine reflexes. Tonic neck reflexes are revealed in the human subject if the cerebral cortex has been extensively damaged. Turning of the patient's head to one side by the examiner initiates a discharge from neck muscles and from receptors around the joints of the upper cervical spine which project to the brain-stem reticular formation. The resulting reflex discharge produces extension of the upper limb on the side to which the head is turned and flexion of the opposite arm. The posture of the upper limb reverses when the head is turned the other way. The lower limbs are little influenced in man.

The position of the head in space exerts a profound influence on spinal cord mechanisms through the otolith organs of the labyrinths and lateral vestibulospinal tracts. Special receptors in the otolith organ of the utricle in the internal ear signal the position of the head in relation to the pull of gravity by means of nerve impulses passing in the vestibular nerve to the lateral vestibular nucleus. The vestibulospinal tracts may then alter the excitability of flexor and extensor tonic reflexes to produce changes in posture. This is seen most clearly in patients who have suffered severe damage to cortex and basal ganglia. When such patients are lifted into the vertical position, their arms usually flex, and the legs extend in the typical 'decorticate' or 'dystonic' posture[7]. If the patient is inverted so the head is downwards, the upper limbs tend to extend and the lower limbs to flex.

Other postural reflexes and the 'righting reflexes' are mediated through mid-brain, basal ganglia and thalamus. The effect on posture of sensory input from the trunk and limbs may be seen on occasions in severely brain-damaged patients. When the patient is lying on one side, the limbs on the lower side may extend and the limbs on the upper side may flex. If the patient is then turned on to the other side, the posture of the limbs changes so that those limbs which were extended become flexed and vice versa.

Cortical reflexes are well recognized in the experimental animal and various hopping and limb placing reactions depend upon the sensorimotor cortex. Excitation of the 'supplementary motor area', which lies on the medial aspect of the frontal lobes rostral to the leg area of the motor cortex, may produce a pattern of flexion and extension in diagonally opposite limbs in man resembling the walking reflexes of an animal[37]. It is not known whether the supplementary motor area participates in the reflex control of posture. All reflex activity is normally held in check by a complex interplay of motor pathways which originate in the pyramidal and extra-pyramidal motor cortex and depend to a great extent upon the basal ganglia and reticular formation. A constant sensory input is necessary for normal motor function and seems to supply a driving force for the sensorimotor cortex, as well as providing the means for precise control of movement through the cerebellum.

Postural reflexes and the motor centres responsible for volitional movement can exert their effects only by action on alpha and gamma motor neurones, the expanded concept of the final common pathway. The most important of the descending pathways influencing 'tone' and postural adjustment are the reticulospinal and vestibulospinal tracts in man. Complementary to their action is that of the pathway which is essential for the production of fine, skilled and repetitive movement in man, the pyramidal or corticospinal tract.

RETICULOSPINAL TRACTS

The reticular formation will be constantly referred to in a discussion of control of the motor system and, in later chapters, in the maintenance of consciousness and awareness. Reticular formation is a

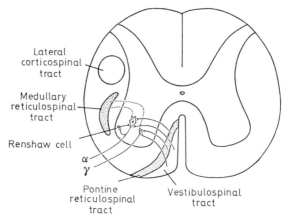

Figure 4.4. Extrapyramidal tracts influencing alpha and gamma motor neurones. Connecting interneurones are not shown for the sake of simplicity. The position of reticulospinal and vestibulospinal pathways is based on studies in the cat by Nyberg–Hansen[34], because their exact position in man is uncertain. The vestibulospinal tract is shown as a crescent since it lies in the ventral segment of the spinal cord in the cervical region and medially along the ventral sulcus in the lumbar region. The pontine reticulospinal tract has a facilitatory action, and the medullary reticulospinal tract has an inhibitory action on the stretch reflex of anti-gravity muscles. Recurrent inhibition of alpha motor neurones by Renshaw cells is discussed in Chapter 5

convenient collective term for the mass of individual neurones which extends throughout the neuraxis from medulla to thalamus and is not grouped in clearly recognizable nuclei. It may be compared with a vague name like 'Milky Way' used to describe a complex heavenly galaxy. It is remarkable that there is sufficient unity of function in the aggregation of nerve cells comprising the reticular

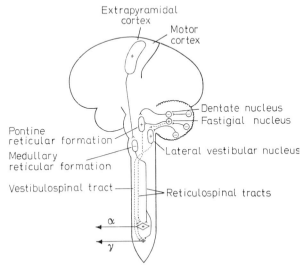

Figure 4.5. Centres and tracts of importance in the control of muscle tone. The medullary reticulospinal tract depends largely upon potentiation from extrapyramidal cortex for its inhibitory effect on the stretch reflex arc of antigravity muscles. Interruption of this corticoreticulospinal pathway at any point along its course will lead to increased tone in these muscles. The pontine reticulospinal tract and vestibulospinal tracts facilitate alpha and gamma motor neurones of antigravity muscles. The cerebellar cortex inhibits the lateral vestibular nucleus directly, as well as inhibiting the dentate and fastigial nuclei, which respectively inhibit and facilitate reticular activity. This leads to a complex situation whereby a cerebellar lesion may increase or decrease alpha and gamma motor neurone activity by a process of disinhibition. In this figure + and — signs indicate the action of one neurone on the next. Further control of the stretch reflex arc takes place at the spinal level by means of facilitatory and inhibitory interneurones, which are indicated in Figure 4.6

formation for it to be regarded as an entity. The reticular formation of the midbrain and thalamus projects diffusely to the cerebral cortex and is essential for the maintenance of consciousness. The pontine and medullary reticular formation projects to the spinal cord through the reticulospinal tracts, which have both facilitatory and inhibitory actions on motor neurones[28]. The reticular formation is thus able to alert the organism via its upstream projection, at the same time setting the stage for activity through its downstream projection. Other parts of the reticular formation are concerned with the regulation of respiration and the vasomotor system.

It is probable that the cerebral cortex, basal ganglia and cerebellum exert most of their effects on the stretch reflex arc through the reticular formation. In the cat, fibres from the same cortical areas as the

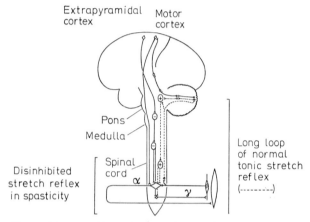

Extrapyramidal cortex   Motor cortex

Pons

Medulla

Disinhibited stretch reflex in spasticity

Spinal cord   α   γ

Long loop of normal tonic stretch reflex (--------)

Figure 4.6. Possible pathway mediating the normal reflex in response to muscle stretch or vibration. It is known that vibration-induced tonic contraction is potentiated from the brain-stem in cat and man. The interrupted lines indicate projection of group Ia afferent fibres rostrally in the dorsal spinocerebellar tract, with hypothetical collaterals (not demonstrated anatomically) impinging on the brain-stem reticular formation to account for the persistence of the phenomenon after ablation of the cerebellum in the cat. In spasticity, the normal graded augmenting tonic contraction is replaced by a crude hyperactive response when the stretch reflex arc is freed from modifying supraspinal influences. In this figure the + and − signs indicate that the whole bulbospinal system is facilitatory or inhibitory

pyramidal tract pass down through the internal capsule to the pontine reticular formation, and, in greater abundance, to the medullary reticular formation. The pontine reticular formation gives rise to an uncrossed reticulospinal tract, which has a facilitatory action on the stretch reflex. Reticulospinal fibres originating in the medulla are both crossed and uncrossed and inhibit the stretch reflex[4]. The origin and course of reticulospinal fibres in man is not well known. It is thought that there is a lateral reticulospinal tract in the lateral columns of the spinal cord, near the corticospinal tract, and a medial reticulospinal tract in the sulco-marginal regions of the anterior columns [33] (*Figure 4.4*).

In spite of the meagreness of anatomical data, the activity of the reticular formation on the stretch reflex arc, particularly the gamma efferent system, has been clearly demonstrated in the cat. Granit and Kaada[16] showed that stimulation of the reticular formation in the hypothalamus, pontine tegmentum and midbrain substantially increased the rate of firing of muscle spindle afferents, and this effect persisted for half a minute or more after stimulation ceased. On the other hand, stimulation of the ventromedial part of the medulla sharply diminished the rate of muscle afferent discharge and often completely suppressed it.

The gamma efferent system may thus be facilitated by the more rostral part of the reticular formation and depressed by the more caudal part in the cat. Whether this applies in detail to man is unknown, but it is probable that the general division into facilitatory and inhibitory reticulospinal pathways is valid for man, and this concept is illustrated in *Figures 4.4, 4.5 and 4.6*.

VESTIBULOSPINAL TRACT

It is probable that the vestibulospinal tract arises from the lateral vestibular nucleus in man, is largely uncrossed, and descends along the periphery of the anterior white columns of the spinal cord[33] (*Figures 4.4 and 4.5*). The vestibular system influences cervical motor neurones by the medial longitudinal fasciculus and both cervical and lumbar motor neurones by reticulospinal pathways as well as by the vestibulospinal tract. The effects of vestibular stimulation are thus bilateral in the cat, and vestibular activity is influenced strongly by position of the head and neck, not only by labyrinthine and cerebellar function, but also indirectly by neck proprioceptors[13].

Stimulation of the vestibular system increases activity of both alpha and gamma motor neurones in the cat. Destruction of the vestibular nuclei abolishes classical decerebrate rigidity.

The vermis of the anterior lobe and part of the posterior lobe of the cerebellum project to the lateral vestibular nucleus directly as well as via the fastigial nucleus (*Figure 4.5*). The cerebellovestibular pathway, as well as the vestibulospinal tract, is arranged somatotopically so that some cerebellar effects may be localized to one part of the spinal cord. Removal or inactivation of the anterior lobe of the cerebellum diminishes excitability of the gamma efferent system, but may nevertheless result in rigidity which is caused by

77

hyperactivity of alpha cells, and has therefore been called 'alpha rigidity'. The vestibulospinal pathways may mediate both types of rigidity, the commonly seen 'gamma' rigidity, operating indirectly through spindle mechanisms, and the rare 'alpha' rigidity. The vestibular nuclei are closely linked with the reticular formation and some vestibular reflexes are produced indirectly through reticulospinal pathways in collaboration with direct vestibulospinal connexions.

Other extrapyramidal tracts

The rubrospinal tract inhibits the gamma system in the cat, but there is no definite evidence that the tract exists in man[33].

The tectospinal tract originates in the superior collicus and after decussating descends in the anterior columns of the cord, mingled with medial vestibulospinal fibres. It is probably responsible for rotary movements of head and trunk in response to visual stimuli[31].

EFFECTS OF EXTRAPYRAMIDAL TRACTS ON THE STRETCH REFLEX

Extrapyramidal pathways terminate on interneurones in the spinal cord, which increase or decrease the excitability of alpha and gamma motor neurones and thus influence the activity of tonic and phasic stretch reflexes. The descending motor fibres which are considered to exert the strongest influence on tone of antigravity muscles in man are the reticulospinal tracts (facilitatory and inhibitory) and the vestibulospinal tract (facilitatory). By means of connexions with the reticular formation, which will be considered later, the extrapyramidal motor cortex, basal ganglia and cerebellum exert control of the stretch reflex and therefore of muscle tone. These influences adjust the sensitivity of the reflex arc and, indirectly, ensure a certain setting of muscle fibre length so that a posture is assumed appropriate for the initiation of voluntary movement. There is a possibility that some voluntary movements may be directed entirely through the 'gamma loop' as are some tonic reflex responses[31]. In any event, this mechanism appears to be the most important in the maintenance of posture against gravity, and the disorder of this system is mainly responsible for most spastic and rigid conditions seen by the clinician.

Tonic stretch reflexes may be temporarily augmented by the Jendrassik manoeuvre (pulling one hand against the grasp of the other) in the same manner as the tendon jerk[29]. This effect depends upon alpha and gamma motor neurones being excited through reticulospinal or propriospinal pathways.

THE MOTOR CORTEX AND PYRAMIDAL TRACT

The pyramidal tract develops in size and complexity as the phylogenetic scale is ascended. Animals such as the bat, rabbit and cow have a short pyramidal tract composed of small axons uniform in calibre. The rat, carnivores and primates possess a long tract, extending through the spinal cord, containing some fibres of large diameter. The greater development of the pyramidal tract in man led to the concept that it is responsible for mediating skilled voluntary movement.

The pyramidal tract in man arises from nerve cells of all sizes in the sensorimotor cortex in the neighbourhood of the central sulcus, with a small contribution from area 6 in front of the motor strip. A few fibres arise from other cortical areas. The course of the tract is well known, and the bulk of its fibres decussate to form the lateral corticospinal tract. In the internal capsule, the fibres of the pyramidal tract are mixed with other fibres descending from the cortex to the reticular formation, substantia nigra and pontine nuclei. At all levels of the nervous system except the medulla, pyramidal fibres are so closely associated with other descending motor tracts that it is almost impossible for any disease to cause a pure pyramidal lesion. This anatomical fact has given rise to the clinical usage of 'upper motor neurone lesion' to cover disturbances of the descending fibre bundle comprising the pyramidal and accompanying extrapyramidal tracts. In the cat, the pyramidal tract terminates on interneurones in the grey matter of the spinal cord but it is now known that many pyramidal fibres make monosynaptic contact with anterior horn cells in monkey and man. Monosynaptic excitation is concentrated particularly on motor neurones serving distal muscle groups, which is presumably important for the cortical control of skilled hand movements[38].

The fibre spectrum of the normal human pyramid in the medulla has two modes of distribution at 1μm and 7μm diameter[41]. Electrical stimulation of the cat pyramid has disclosed two waves of electrical activity, indicating two fibre groups of different conduction velocity which have somewhat different properties[3] (*Figure 4.7*). Electrical activity from these two groups may be recorded from the pyramids when the motor cortex is stimulated[25], although the response is complicated by the repetitive firing of cortical neurones[36]. Stimulation of the medullary pyramid induces antidromic impulses in the

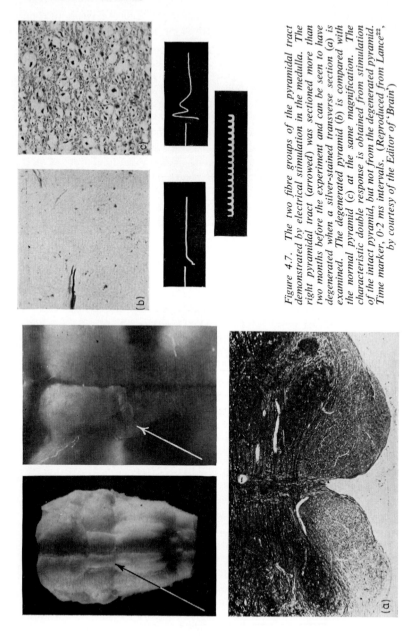

Figure 4.7. The two fibre groups of the pyramidal tract demonstrated by electrical stimulation in the medulla. The right pyramidal tract (arrowed) was sectioned more than two months before the experiment and can be seen to have degenerated when a silver-stained transverse section (a) is examined. The degenerated pyramid (b) is compared with the normal pyramid (c) at the same magnification. The characteristic double response is obtained from stimulation of the intact pyramid, but not from the degenerated pyramid. Time marker, 0·2 ms intervals. (Reproduced from Lance[22], by courtesy of the Editor of 'Brain')

pyramidal tract, which discharge cell bodies in the motor cortex. The presence of two groups of fibres has been confirmed in this way by recording from the white matter[42] and cortex[43]. The two groups have also been traced down to the lumbar segments of the cat cord[21].

Evarts[11] has shown in recordings made from the unanaesthetized monkey that pyramidal neurones of high axonal conduction velocity are active mainly during movement, while those of low conduction velocity tend to discharge tonically. Evarts also demonstrated that pairs of adjacent neurones in the motor cortex discharged reciprocally during voluntary movement. The difficulty of simulating voluntary movement by artificial methods is thus explained as the area of cortex stimulated may well contain neurones influencing antagonistic muscle groups.

Repetitive stimulation of the pyramidal tract first facilitates 3-neurone arcs (which generally serve flexor or protective reflexes), followed by facilitation of the 2-neurone stretch reflex arc[27]. Granit and Kaada[16] produced transient acceleration of muscle spindle discharges by stimulation of the medullary pyramid. The same spindle could be activated from the contralateral motor area. Stimulation of the motor cortex generally caused gamma efferent activity at a lower threshold than alpha activity, although it must be remembered that the animals were under anaesthesia. Gernandt and Gilman[13] found that repetitive stimulation of the motor cortex in the cat enhanced the monosynaptic reflex arc in the spinal cord, and that this was followed by a profound depression lasting about a minute. This depressant effect persisted after the pyramidal tract was sectioned in the medulla, suggesting that it was mediated by collaterals passing to the reticular formation. Stimulation of the medullary pyramid, on the other hand, elicited a facilitation of the monosynaptic arc for a minute or more without any phase of depression. This finding of facilitatory effects alone from the medullary pyramid fits in with the hypotonic paresis which has been generally reported as a result of experimental section of the pyramidal tract. Some observers have noticed a slight increase in extensor tone on the affected side after pyramidotomy, particularly when the animal was suspended above the ground, but there has never been any indication of the spasticity which is seen after extensive lesions of the motor cortex or lesions of the internal capsule. Spasticity from cortical lesions is the result of interruption of fibres passing from the motor cortex and 'extrapyramidal' cortex in front of the motor strip to the basal ganglia and inhibitory reticular formation in the medulla which suppresses the stretch reflex arc through the inhibitory reticulospinal tract[28] (*See Figure 4.5*).

Gernandt and Gilman also observed that the first volley discharged from anterior horn cells in response to stimulation of the motor cortex disappeared after section of the pyramid. Activity still followed in anterior roots but the response was of longer latency and lower amplitude. This accords with earlier descriptions of the defect in fine skilled movement in animals whose pyramidal tract had been sectioned, with the preservation of more simple stereo-typed movement. Tower[44] found that stimulation of the cat motor cortex produced relaxation of extensor tonus whether or not the pyramidal tract was severed, but that small transient movements appeared only when the pyramidal pathway was intact.

Pyramidal section has little effect on a cat's motor performance. Cortical reflexes, such as hopping and placing reactions, are lost and the cat has difficulty with skilled flexion movements on the affec-ted side, but it can run around on firm ground with no apparent disability. The effect of pyramidal damage is greater in higher animals. Gait is affected in monkeys, the animals dragging the affec-ted limb. There is a hypotonic hemiparesis with sluggish deep reflexes, and a deficit of accurate movements. Abdominal and cremasteric reflexes are diminished, and protective flexor reflexes are absent[45]. In the chimpanzee an extensor plantar response is observed after pyramidal section[46]. There have been a number of reports of natural lesions in man which affected chiefly the pyramidal tract. Since the cause of such lesions is usually cerebral vascular disease, there is always an element of uncertainty as to the extent to which other structures are involved. A patient recently reported, in whom the pyramidal tract was interrupted by a cyst at the pontomedullary junction, suffered a hemiplegia which was at first flaccid but later became spastic[5].

THE TONIC STRETCH REFLEX IN MAN

In Chapter 3, deep muscle reflexes ('tendon jerks') were shown to be phasic reflexes mediated by the monosynaptic arc in response to a sudden vibration or stretch of the muscle spindle. If a standard physiotherapy vibrator with a reasonably large baseplate is applied to a muscle belly, or a vibrator with a small applicator is held against a muscle tendon, continued vibration will induce a slow tonic contraction in the appropriate muscle [6, 17, 23].

This tonic contraction is the result of vibration of muscle spindles inducing activity in group Ia afferents[2, 8], thus acting as a sustained stretch stimulus. It therefore serves as a model for the study of the tonic stretch reflex in man. Like a phasic stretch reflex, this tonic reflex requires integrity of the monosynaptic arc, but additional supraspinal reinforcement is necessary for its full development. Matthews[30] has shown that the reflex may be obtained in the decerebrate cat and that it persists after ablation of the cerebellum but disappears 2–30 minutes after the spinal cord is sectioned. In man, the reflex is diminished on the side of an upper neurone lesion or a cerebellar disturbance and is altered in character below the level of spinal section in a paraplegic or quadriplegic patient[9, 18, 24]. It is probable that vibration-induced tonic contraction is normally facilitated and regulated by a spino-bulbo-spinal relay[40] which is influenced by the motor cortex and cerebellum (*see Figure 4.6*).

The tonic contraction evoked by muscle vibration in man increases over a period of about thirty seconds until it reaches a plateau.

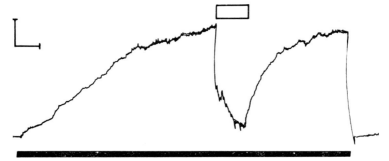

Figure 4.8. Voluntary suppression of vibration-induced tonic contraction. Recording of force exerted on a force-transducer at the ankle, when the quadriceps was vibrated while the subject was lying down, with the leg flexed at the knee over the end of an examination couch. The open bar indicates the period during which the subject was asked to relax the quadriceps. When the subject's attention was distracted, the tonic contraction returned rapidly to its previous level. Calibration: vertical 0·4 kg; horizontal 10 s. (Reproduced from de Gail, Lance and Neilson[6] by courtesy of the Editor of J. Neurol. Neurosurg. Psychiat.)

It may be inhibited voluntarily but as soon as the attention of the subject is distracted, the contraction builds up again (*Figure 4.8*). If tonic contraction is in progress and an antagonistic muscle is vibrated, the initial contraction is inhibited and gives place to a tonic contraction in the antagonist (*Figure 4.9*). The progressive augmenting nature of the tonic contraction in man, which is not seen in the anaesthetized or decerebrate animal, may depend upon the cerebellum which receives a substantial contribution from group Ia afferent fibres and which is known to facilitate both alpha and gamma motor neurones[19]. Gamma activation, by contracting muscle spindles, makes their receptors more sensitive to stretch

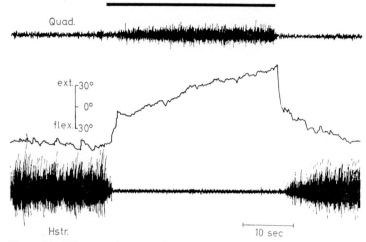

Figure 4.9. Vibration of reciprocally innervated muscles with limb unrestrained (isotonic contraction). Vibration of hamstrings is continued throughout, with flexion of the knee initially (middle tracing) and EMG activity being recorded from the hamstrings muscle bellies (lower tracing). When a second vibrator is applied to the quadriceps muscle (solid bar at top), tonic contraction in hamstrings is inhibited, with return of the leg to the neutral position before a tonic contraction starts in quadriceps (upper EMG tracing). At the end of quadriceps vibration, contraction of hamstrings resumes. (Reproduced from Lance, de Gail and Neilson[24] by courtesy of the Editor of J. Neurol. Neurosurg. Psychiat.)

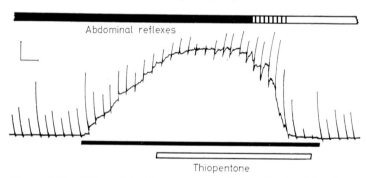

Figure 4.10. Effect of barbiturate anaesthesia on vibration-induced tonic contraction. While a tonic contraction was produced by vibration of the quadriceps in a normal subject, the knee jerk was elicited at 5-second intervals and the abdominal reflexes tested repeatedly. Following the intravenous injections of thiopentone, the tonic contraction and abdominal reflexes disappeared while tendon jerks persisted[6]. Recording of force exerted at the ankle as in Figure 4.8. Calibration: vertical 0·4 kg; horizontal 10 s. (Reproduced by courtesy of the Editor of J. Neurol Neurosurg. Psychiat.)

84

or vibration and could thus augment tonic contraction (*see Figure 4.6*).

The tonic reflex, being dependent upon asynchronous bombardment of anterior horn cells, requires the participation of supraspinal structures to provide a 'starter function' in initiating muscle contraction and to potentiate alpha cell activity while the contraction is in progress. The sensitivity of the alpha cell to temporal summation of asynchronous impulses is impaired by hypoxia, anaesthesia[1], or drugs such as barbiturates, diazepam (Valium) and benztropine methanesulphonate (Cogentin), which block tonic contraction but not the phasic reflexes resulting from synchronous afferent volleys (*Figures 4.10, 4.11*).

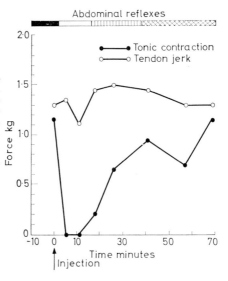

Figure 4.11. Effect of drugs used in the treatment of spasticity on vibration-induced tonic contraction. The intravenous injection of diazepam or the experimental drug Ciba-28,882-Ba, abolishes the tonic contraction and abdominal reflexes, without significantly affecting tendon jerks[6]. (Reproduced by courtesy of the Editor of J. Neurol. Neurosurg. Psychiat.)

The vibration-induced tonic contraction in man has characteristics different from those of spasticity or extrapyramidal rigidity. It is more variable in latency and intensity than the abnormal tonic stretch reflexes found in these conditions and is abolished rather than augmented by the application of sudden stretch to the muscle. Vibration-induced tonic contraction is a physiological reaction found in its most complete form in normal subjects and may be considered as a means of testing the pathway for tonic stretch reflexes in intact man. The reaction is usually diminished in patients with upper motor neurone lesions, but in those patients who show the increased tonic stretch reflexes of spasticity, the normal augmenting muscle contraction in response to vibration is replaced by an extensor thrust. If the limb of a spastic patient is in such a position that

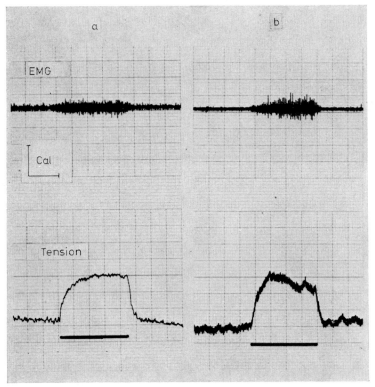

Figure 4.12. Comparison of the vibration-induced tonic contraction in spastic man with that of the anaesthetized or decerebrated cat. (a) EMG and force of contraction evoked in gastrocnemius-soleus of the pentobarbitone-anaesthetized cat by vibration of tendo achillis at 200/second (black bar). The pattern of contraction is similar in the decerebrate animal. (b) EMG and force of contraction evoked in gastrocnemius-soleus of a patient with spastic paraparesis resulting from angioma of the thoracic spinal cord. The frequency of vibration (black bar) was limited to 100/second, since higher frequencies produced clonus. The sudden increase in muscle tension is quite unlike the progressively augmenting contraction seen in intact man. Calibration: vertical, EMG (a) 0·5 mV (b) 0·25 mV; force (a and b) 0·25 kg; horizontal, 5 s. (From Burke, Gillies and Lance; unpublished.)

increased resistance to stretch can be palpated, the effect of vibration is to initiate a muscle contraction of rapid onset which ceases immediately vibration stops, quite unlike the slowly augmenting reflex in normal subjects (*Figure 4.12*). Hagbarth and Eklund[18] commented that reaction in the spastic patients resembled the contraction induced by vibration in Matthews' decerebrate cats. If the limb of a spastic patient is moved into a position of flaccidity, that is, flexed to the point where the clasp-knife reaction has taken place and there is no palpable stretch reflex, then vibration of muscle will not evoke any tonic contraction. Changes in the nature of vibration-induced contraction therefore run parallel to those of the tonic

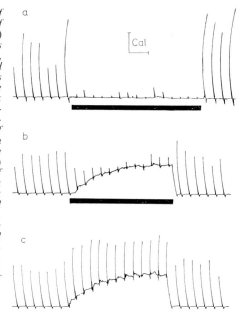

Figure 4.13. Suppression of tendon jerks by vibration of the appropriate muscle. (a) Vibration of the quadriceps muscle in a normal subject, with knee jerks elicited every 5 seconds. Knee jerks are depressed during the period of vibration (black bar) even without the development of a tonic contraction. (b) Suppression of knee jerks accompanying a tonic contraction induced by vibration (black bar). (c) Voluntary contraction of quadriceps in same subject as (b). The knee jerk is not depressed during the period of voluntary contraction. Calibration: vertical 0·4 kg for (a), 0·6 kg for (b) and (c). horizontal 10 s. (Reproduced from de Gail, Lance and Neilson[6] by courtesy of the Editor of J. Neurol. Neurosurg. Psychiat.)

stretch reflex, and demonstrate clearly the difference between the normal and spastic state. This implies that the tonic stretch reflexes of spasticity are not simply exaggerated normal responses, but employ only part of the normal pathway, being deprived of the supraspinal connexions required for the normal graded reflex contraction.

It might be imagined that vibration of muscle which induced activity in group Ia afferents would augment phasic as well as tonic mechanisms and that deep reflexes would be increased. In fact, the reverse occurs and phasic reflexes are progressively suppressed by vibration[6, 14, 23] (*Figure 4.13*). The apparent paradox of phasic reflexes being suppressed while a tonic reflex was elicited suggested the possibility of two different types of motor neurone which were affected differentially by the reflex effects of vibration, since some motor neurones have exhibited predominantly tonic or phasic properties in the experimental animal[15]. This concept was tested in man by recording single motor units in muscle during a phasic response (H reflex) and a tonic response (vibration-induced contraction)[24]. Some units were found which participated in both tonic

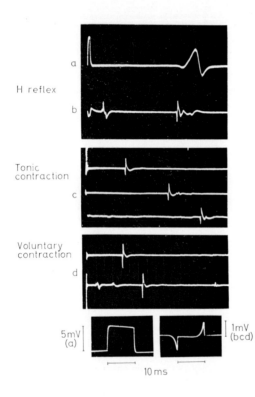

H reflex

Tonic contraction

Voluntary contraction

5mV
(a)

1mV
(bcd)

10 ms

Figure 4.14. Single motor unit participation in tonic and phasic reflexes. (a) An EMG recorded from the soleus muscle by surface electrodes, following single shock to medial popliteal nerve, showing the H reflex. (b) An EMG recorded simultaneously through a bipolar needle electrode, showing participation of a single motor unit in the H reflex. (c) Three random samples (50 ms duration) recorded from a needle electrode in the same position during tonic contraction of soleus muscle induced by vibration of tendo achillis. A single motor unit is recorded, which has the same appearance as that recorded during elicitation of the H reflex. (d) Two random samples recorded from a needle electrode during slight voluntary contraction of the soleus muscle, without the position of the electrode being altered. The same motor unit is again recorded. (Reproduced from Lance, de Gail and Neilson[24], by courtesy of the Editor of J. Neurol. Neurosurg. Psychiat.)

and phasic reactions as well as taking part in normal voluntary contraction (*Figure 4.14*). Since the same motor neurone may mediate both types of reaction, how can phasic reflexes be suppressed by vibration while a tonic contraction develops? Hunt[20] demonstrated that stretching a muscle reduced the size of the monosynaptic reflex response in the same muscle. Recent work in our laboratory[14] has shown that vibration of muscle, stimulating stretch receptors, suppresses the monosynaptic reflex by a process of presynaptic inhibition, that is, the terminals of group Ia afferents become depolarized by interneurones and are unable to transmit afferent volleys directly to motor neurones. This finding means that the initiation of tonic reflexes by stretch or vibration has to overcome presynaptic inhibition of the monosynaptic arc, either by a process of temporal summation of impulses or by switching of activity from monosynaptic to polysynaptic pathways. The dependence of normal regulation of muscle tone upon a long supraspinal loop explains why changes in muscle tone and tendon jerks need not run parallel. The pathway mediating tonic reflexes may be influenced above the segmental level independently of changes in excitability of alpha and gamma motor neurones which alone determine the briskness of the tendon jerk.

Considering the present evidence there does not appear to be any need to postulate separate tonic and phasic anterior horn cells in man. The motor neurone may react phasically if it is presented with a synchronous afferent volley. When the afferent barrage is asynchronous from muscle stretch or an artificial stimulus such as vibration, alpha motor neurones have to be raised to an adequate level of excitability in order to respond with sustained tonic discharge. The normal mechanism for this appears to be the alerting response mediated through descending pathways such as the facilitatory reticulospinal tract. It may be thrown into activity by its cortical connexions in preparation for voluntary movement, or by the spino-bulbo-spinal pathway as a part of tonic reflexes initiated by stretch or vibration. When descending motor pathways are damaged at any level from cortex to spinal cord, the normal mechanism for the adjustment of muscle tone appropriate to movement is lost, and the tonic stretch reflex arc becomes 'short-circuited' in a state of facilitation, which is termed spasticity (*Figure 4.6*).

THE NORMAL CONTROL OF MOVEMENT

Under normal circumstances in a relaxed subject standing at ease, the stretch reflex is inactive since the body is balanced over the centre of gravity[10]. If the subject is anxious, if the body is slightly displaced from a neutral balanced position, if a posture is to be maintained against gravity, or if a voluntary movement starts in one part of the body, stretch reflexes become active. This effect is mediated through the gamma efferent system via the reticulospinal pathways, the downstream alerting mechanism. Maintenance of posture and the alteration of posture in response to head position or neck movement is mediated through both vestibulospinal and reticulospinal pathways.

The antigravity posture may be interrupted by protective segmental reflexes which cause withdrawal of a limb by a flexion movement. In addition, intersegmental reflexes impose rhythmical patterns of flexion and extension upon segmental organization by means of propriospinal fibres to produce walking and running movements and these may be influenced by the supplementary motor area on the medial aspect of the frontal cortex. Certain hopping and placing reactions are mediated by a long reflex arc, with an afferent limb of proprioceptive fibres reaching up to the cerebral cortex and producing an efferent motor discharge which alters posture. Some primitive reflexes normally suppressed by the cortex may be seen in the adult only when brain damage has removed this controlling influence. Superimposed upon spinal and supraspinal reflexes are the effects of extrapyramidal and pyramidal tracts whose activity modifies muscle tone and produces volitional movement.

The initiation of movement from the motor cortex requires corticofugal pathways other than the pyramidal tract. Cortico-rubrospinal fibres are important in the cat, and corticoreticulospinal fibres probably serve this function in man. Extrapyramidal pathways may produce fairly complex movement as well as stereotyped flexor or extensor synergies in which all flexor or extensor muscles of a limb act together.

The pyramidal tract probably has both tonic and phasic functions. Here the term phasic is extended to cover transient movements and is not restricted to a synchronous motor neurone volley. The tonic function facilitates flexor mechanisms in the lower limb and, to a lessor extent, extensor mechanisms in the upper limb, which results in a posture suitable for action involving that side of the body. The phasic function is the mediation of skilled movement, mostly involving distal muscles. In the cat and other animals which do not move the digits independently, the pyramidal tract influences motor neurones through internuncial cells. As the evolutionary scale is ascended, the pyramidal tract acquires monosynaptic contact with motor neurones, thus permitting direct control of muscles used in skilled movement.

Flexor reflexes are uninhibited in the infant but are brought under supraspinal control during the first year of life so that the lower limbs may be maintained in the extended posture necessary for standing. The vestibulospinal tract is probably the most important in determining the antigravity standing posture. As the child learns to walk, controlled flexion movements, mediated chiefly by the pyramidal tract, become superimposed on the standing posture. In the adult, movement is regulated by the motor cortex through extrapyramidal as well as pyramidal pathways, the former co-operating with the tonic function of the pyramidal tract in determining posture by contraction of proximal muscles, while the phasic component of the pyramidal tract is responsible for fine distal movements of the limb.

SUMMARY

Tonic stretch reflexes are of greater physiological and clinical significance than phasic stretch reflexes. They comprise the 'muscle tone' of the clinician and determine posture. Tonic stretch reflexes may be studied in man by vibration of muscle which stimulates muscle spindles in the same manner as stretch, thus producing a tonic contraction of the muscle vibrated. This physiological reaction is augmented and regulated by supraspinal mechanisms which are in turn influenced by the motor cortex and cerebellum. Such influences may alter muscle tone independently of phasic reflexes (tendon jerks), which depend solely upon the monosynaptic arc. It is probable that the same motor neurones mediate both tonic and phasic mechanisms in man. The initiation of tonic reflexes is usually accompanied by depression of the monosynaptic arc through a process of presynaptic inhibition. When the upper motor neurone is damaged, the normal tonic reflex mechanism is short-circuited and the monosynaptic arc is dominated by facilitatory spinal mechanisms, producing the clinical state known as spasticity.

Internuncial cell systems in the spinal cord may exert facilitatory or inhibitory effects upon both tonic and phasic action of alpha motor neurones. Both alpha and gamma motor neurones may also be influenced by propriospinal pathways, the pyramidal tract, inhibitory and facilitatory reticulospinal tracts, and vestibulospinal tract. The vestibulospinal tract has a facilitatory action upon the motor neurones of antigravity muscles, predominantly upper limb flexors and lower limb extensors when man is in the erect position. The pyramidal tract probably has both tonic and phasic functions, the former favouring extension of the upper limbs and flexion of the lower limbs. Extrapyramidal pathways regulate alpha or gamma bias, altering the excitability of alpha and gamma motor neurones to both spinal and supraspinal stimulation. Extrapyramidal tracts may mediate some movements as well as controlling posture. The distinction between pyramidal and extrapyramidal pathways is anatomical, not physiological, since their cortical origins overlap and their action at spinal cord level is complementary in the control of muscle tone and movement. The acquisition of independent movements of the digits as the evolutionary scale is ascended is accompanied by the development of direct monosynaptic control of motor neurones by the pyramidal tract, thus permitting skilled movement of distal muscles.

REFERENCES

[1] Alvord, E. C. and Fuortes, M. G. F. (1953). 'Reflex activity of extensor motor units following muscular afferent excitation.' *J. Physiol.* **122**, 302–321

[2] Bianconi, R. and Van der Meulen, J. P. (1963). 'The response to vibration of the end organs of mammalian muscle spindles.' *J. Neurophysiol.* **26**, 177–190

[3] Bishop, P. O., Jeremy, D. and Lance, J. W. (1953). 'Properties of pyramidal tract.' *J. Neurophysiol.* **16**, 537–550

[4] Brodal, A. (1962). 'Spasticity—anatomical aspects.' *Acta neurol. scand.* **38**, Suppl. 3, 9–40

[5] Brown, W. J. and Fang, H. C. H. (1961). 'Spastic hemiplegia in man. Lack of flaccidity in lesion of pyramidal tract.' *Neurology, Minneap.* **11**, 829–835

[6] de Gail, P., Lance, J. W. and Neilson, P. D. (1966). 'Differential effects on tonic and phasic reflex mechanisms produced by vibration of muscles in man.' *J. Neurol. Neurosurg. Psychiat.* **29**, 1–11

[7] Denny-Brown, D. (1962). *The Basal Ganglia and their Relation to Disorders of Movement*, p. 29. London; Oxford University Press

[8] Echlin, F. and Fessard, A. (1938). 'Synchronized impulse discharges from receptors in the deep tissue in response to a vibrating stimulus.' *J. Physiol. Lond.* **93**, 312–334

[9] Eklund, G. and Hagbarth, K-E. (1966). 'Normal variability of tonic vibration reflexes in man.' *Exp. Neurol.* **16**, 80–92

[10] Eldred, E. (1960). 'Posture and locomotion.' In *American Physiological Society Handbook of Physiology*. Ed. by J. Field. Sect. 1, Vol. 2, pp. 1074–5. Baltimore; Williams and Wilkins

[11] Evarts, E. V. (1965). 'Relation of discharge frequencies to conduction velocity in pyramidal tract neurons.' *J. Neurophysiol.* **28**, 216–228

[12] Gelfan, S. and Tarlov, I. M. (1959). 'Interneurons and rigidity of spinal origin.' *J. Physiol. Lond.* **146**, 594–617

[13] Gernandt, B. O. and Gilman, S. (1960). 'Interactions between vestibular, pyramidal and cortically evoked extrapyramidal activities.' *J. Neurophysiol.* **23**, 516–533

[14] Gillies, J. D., Tassinari, C., Neilson, P. D. and Lance, J. W. (1969). 'Presynaptic inhibition of the monosynaptic reflex, by vibration.' *J. Physiol., Lond.* **25**, 329–339

[15] Granit, R., Henatsch, H. D. and Steg. G. (1956). 'Tonic and phasic ventral horn cells differentiated by post-tetanic potentiation in cat extensors.' *Acta. physiol. scand.* **37**, 114–126

[16] Granit, R. and Kaada, B. R. (1952). 'Influence of stimulation of central nervous structures on muscle spindles in cat.' *Acta. physiol. scand.* **27**, 130–160

[17] Hagbarth, K-E. and Eklund, G. (1965). 'Motor effects of vibratory muscle stimuli in man.' In *Proceedings of the First Nobel Symposium, Stockholm, 1964*, pp. 177–186. Ed. by Granit, R. Stockholm; Almqvist and Wiksell

[18] Hagbarth, K-E. and Eklund, G. (1968). 'The effects of muscle vibration in spasticity, rigidity and cerebellar disorders.' *J. Neurol. Neurosurg. Psychiat.* **81**, 207–213

[19] Henatsch, H. D., Manni, E., Wilson, J. H. and Dow, R. S. (1964). 'Linked and independent responses of tonic alpha and gamma hindlimb motoneurons to deep cerebellar stimulation.' *J. Neurophysiol.* **27**, 172–192

[20] Hunt, C. C. (1952). 'The effect of stretch receptors from muscle on the discharge of motoneurones.' *J. Physiol. Lond.* **117**, 359–379

[21] Lance, J. W. (1954). 'Pyramidal tract in spinal cord of cat.' *J. Neurophysiol.* **17**, 253–270

[22] Lance, J. W. (1954). 'Behaviour of pyramidal axons following section.' *Brain* **77**, 314–324

[23] Lance, J. W. (1965). 'The mechanism of reflex irradiation.' *Proc. Aust. Ass. Neurol.* **3**, 77–81

[24] Lance, J. W., de Gail, P. and Neilson, P. D. (1966). 'Tonic and phasic spinal cord mechanisms in man.' *J. Neurol. Neurosurg. Psychiat.* **29**, 535–544

[25] Lance, J. W. and Manning, R. L. (1954). 'Origin of the pyramidal tract in the cat.' *J. Physiol. Lond.* **124**, 385–399

[26] Languth, H. W., Teasdall, R. D. and Magladery, J. W. (1952). 'Electrophysiological studies of reflex activity in patients with lesions of the nervous sytem. III. Motoneurone excitability following afferent nerve volleys in patients with rostrally adjacent spinal cord damage.' *Bull. Johns Hopkins Hosp.* **91**, 257–266

[27] Lloyd, D. P. C. (1941). 'The spinal mechanisms of the pyramidal system in cats.' *J. Neurophysiol.* **4**, 525–546

[28] Magoun, H. W. and Rhines, R. (1947). *Spasticity: The Stretch Reflex and Extrapyramidal Systems*. Springfield, Illinois; Thomas

[29] Mark, R. F. (1963). 'Tonic stretch reflexes in the calf muscles of normal human subjects.' *Nature, Lond.* **199**, 50–52

[30] Matthews, P. B. C. (1966). 'The reflex excitation of the soleus muscle of the decerebrate cat caused by vibration applied to its tendon.' *J. Physiol. Lond.* **184**, 450–472

[31] Merton, P. A. (1953). 'Speculations on the servo-control of movement.' In *The Spinal Cord. Ciba Foundation Symposium.* Ed. by Wolstenholme. London; Churchill

[32] Murayama, S. and Smith, C. M. (1965). 'Rigidity of hind limbs of cats produced by occlusion of spinal cord blood supply.' *Neurology, Minneap.* **15**, 565–577

[33] Nathan, P. W. and Smith, M. C. (1955). 'Long descending tracts in man. I. Review of present knowledge.' *Brain* **78**, 248–303

[34] Nyberg-Hansen, R. (1966). 'Functional organization of descending supraspinal fibre systems to the spinal cord.' *Ergebn., Anat. EntwGesch.* **39**, 1–48

[35] Paillard, J. (1955). *Réflexes et Régulations d'Origine Proprioceptive Chez l'Homme.* Paris; Arnette

[36] Paton, H. D. and Amassian, V. E. (1960). 'The pyramidal tract: its excitation and functions.' In *American Physiological Society Handbook of Physiology*. Ed. by J. Field, Sect. 1, Vol. 2, pp. 837–861. Baltimore; Williams and Wilkins

[37] Penfield, W. and Jasper, H. (1954). *Epilepsy and the Functional Anatomy of the Human Brain*. Boston; Little, Brown

[38] Phillips, C. G. (1967). 'Corticomotoneuronal organization.' *Archs Neurol*. **17**, 188–195

[39] Rushworth, G., Lishman, W. A., Hughes, J. T. and Oppenheimer, D. R. (1961). 'Intense rigidity of the arms due to isolation of motoneurones by a spinal tumour.' *J. Neurol. Neurosurg. Psychiat*. **24**, 132–142

[40] Shimamura, M. and Akert, K.(1965). 'Peripheral nervous relations of propriospinal and spino-bulbo-spinal reflex systems.' *Jap. J. Physiol*. **15**, 638–647

[41] Szentàgothai–Schimert, J. (1965). 'Bedeutung des Faserkalibers und der Markscheidendicke im Zentralnervensystem.' *Z. Anat. Entwgesch*. **3**, 201–223

[42] Takahashi, K. (1965). 'Slow and fast groups of pyramidal tract cells and their respective membrane properties.' *J. Neurophysiol*. **28**, 908–924

[43] Towe, A. L., Patton, H. D. and Kennedy, T. T. (1963). 'Properties of the pyramidal system in the cat.' *Expl. Neurol*. **8**, 220–239

[44] Tower, S. S. (1935). 'The dissociation of cortical excitation from cortical inhibition by pyramid section, and the syndrome of that lesion in the cat.' *Brain* **58**, 238–255

[45] Tower, S. S. (1940). 'Pyramidal lesion in the monkey.' *Brain* **63**, 36–90

[46] Tower, S. S. (1949). 'The pyramidal tract.' In *The Precentral Motor Cortex*, pp. 149–172. Ed. by P. Bucy. Univ. of Illinois Press

5—Disordered Control of Motor Neurones

Motor neurones may be spurred into action by spinal reflexes or by the descending motor pathways mediating voluntary movement. In either event, anterior horn cells must discharge at a frequency just sufficient to produce a change of posture or skilled movement. The rate of discharge must be enough to generate a muscle contraction of suitable force for the task and a balance must be maintained between contraction of agonist and antagonist for smooth performance. The discharge must be as nearly asynchronous as possible to avoid oscillatory movements of the limb. Some discussion of the normal regulation of motor neurone activity is necessary before proceeding further with the mechanisms of tremor, spasticity and rigidity.

FREQUENCY CONTROL OF MOTOR NEURONES

In the decerebrate cat, motor neurones participating in lumbar spinal reflexes may discharge at frequencies of 5–90 per second[1], but usually discharge at about 10 per second irrespective of the frequency of afferent activity[2]. Postural muscles, such as soleus, may develop 90 per cent of their maximum tension with a discharge frequency of only 15 per second in the cat[4]. In man, motor units have not been observed to discharge more rapidly than 10 per second during the tonic contraction produced by muscle vibration[17], although they may reach rates of 40–50 per second in voluntary contraction.

In cats, distinctive tonic and phasic patterns of motor neurone activity have been described, the tonic discharge being of low frequency and well sustained, whereas phasic activity is characterized by transient bursts of high frequency impulses. There is no evidence for tonic and phasic cells being distinct in man and it appears that the same alpha motor neurones may respond in tonic or phasic fashion depending on the degree of synchrony of afferent impulses, and on the amount of supraspinal reinforcement. Alpha cells may be activated reflexly by group Ia afferent neurones through the mono-synaptic arc and also by interneurones or propriospinal fibres mediating reflexes originating in other segments of the spinal cord. They may also be discharged by the descending motor pathways as a part of high-level reflex activity or voluntary movement. The ease with which alpha motor neurones discharge in response to afferent impulses depends upon the sum total of facilitatory and inhibitory influences active upon the cell at that particular time. A steady inflow of impulses from group Ia afferents as a result of muscle stretch (or spindle contraction from gamma efferent activity) which is not sufficient to discharge the neurone reflexly, may be enough to lower its threshold of excitation. Stimulation of Golgi tendon organs by muscle contraction or excessive tension causes a discharge of Ib afferents which diminishes the activity of motor neurones supplying that muscle. There may be excitatory or inhibitory influences from contralateral afferents, intersegmental reflexes and spinal cord internuncial cells, all of which affect the threshold of discharge of the alpha motor neurone. In addition, the activity of internuncial cells is regulated by descending motor pathways. All polysynaptic reflex paths to alpha motor neurones can be facilitated by the cortex through the corticospinal tract, whereas most polysynaptic pathways, such as those from afferents serving flexor reflexes and from Golgi tendon organs, can be presynaptically inhibited from the brain-stem, or inhibited through post-synaptic action on interneurones[22]. Such inhibition is absent in the spinal animal. These observations help to explain why flexion movements are impaired with cortico-spinal lesions, why flexor reflexes are suppressed in decerebrate patients, and why flexor spasms may predominate in patients with spinal lesions.

There is another inhibitory mechanism which is important in preventing rapid firing of the motor neurone and prohibiting repetitive firing in response to a single stimulus. This is 'recurrent inhibition' by the Renshaw cell. Each alpha axon gives off a collateral before it leaves the spinal grey matter which makes synaptic contact with a small cell, known as the Renshaw cell (*see Figure 4.4*). The Renshaw cell then projects back on to the alpha motor neurone to prevent its discharging again for up to 100 ms.[9, 34]. This process of recurrent inhibition is more apparent on the tonic activity of motor neurones. There is evidence that the Renshaw cell system is under supraspinal control[8]. Should the Renshaw cells become hyperactive, the maximal discharge frequency of anterior horn cells would drop and the force of muscle contraction could diminish. Conversely, suppression of Renshaw cell action would increase the discharge frequency of alpha cells and tend to produce a tetanic contraction of muscle like that seen in tonic seizures. Synchronization of Renshaw cell activity could produce simultaneous cycles of excitability and depression in all tonic alpha motor neurones which would evoke a tremor rhythm with beats appearing simultaneously in flexors and extensors, agonist and antagonist. It so happens that such synchronous activity is the pattern of physiological tremor rhythm.

It would be tempting to assume that the tendency of a motor neurone to discharge tonically at about 10 per second when stimulated in an asynchronous or random fashion is the result of Renshaw cell activity, were it not for the demonstration by Redman and Lampard[28] that the discharge rate is unaltered after blocking the activity of Renshaw cells. The limiting of frequency response during tonic discharge is apparently inherent in the afferent terminals impinging on the motor neurone.

PHYSIOLOGICAL OR ACTION TREMOR

Normal subjects have no tremor at rest but on maintaining a posture such as holding out the arms, or on performing a strong muscular contraction, a fine tremor will become apparent. This can usually be seen, particularly if a sheet of paper is placed over the outstretched fingers, and can easily be recorded by a suitable transducer such as an accelerometer. The rate of physiological tremor is about 6 c/s in young children, increasing with maturity to 8–12 c/s and decreases again with advancing years[24]. The rhythm is not obvious in an electromyogram (EMG) unless the individual has an unusually conspicuous tremor, or is contracting a muscle toward the limit of strength. The fluctuations of muscle potential are often obscured by the high voltage 'interference pattern' of muscle contraction, consisting of the superimposed potentials of many motor units. However, the rhythm can be detected in the EMG of many normal subjects[21] and it becomes discernible on EMG recordings (as well as being clinically apparent) in the following conditions:

Anxiety states	Uraemia
Fatigue	Hepatic pre-coma
Hangover	Thyrotoxicosis
Chronic alcoholism	
Hypoglycaemia	Muscular weakness, for example,
Hypercapnia	following poliomyelitis
Hereditary 'simple' tremor	Parkinson's disease

It is diminished or absent in myxoedema and in some patients with lesions in the vicinity of the internal capsule. The reduction of action tremor in myxoedema may be the result of the protraction of the time taken for a muscle twitch. This slowing of muscle contraction and relaxation is responsible for the long duration of deep muscle reflexes in myxoedema[27] and may smooth out synchrony of central action by failing to follow a tremor rhythm.

ACTION TREMOR AND ALTERNATING TREMOR IN PARKINSON'S DISEASE

The exaggerated physiological tremor or 'action tremor' of Parkinson's disease must not be confused with the slower alternating tremor which usually appears later in the same condition. Action tremor

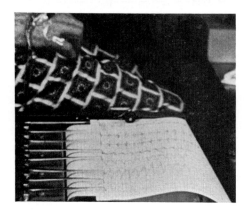

Figure 5.1. Alternating tremor in Parkinson's disease. Surface electrodes attached to biceps, triceps, wrist flexors and wrist extensors demonstrate that beats of tremor alternate between antagonistic muscles while the limb is at rest, imparting a to-and-fro movement to the hand at 3–7 c/s, recorded by an accelerometer in the bottom tracing

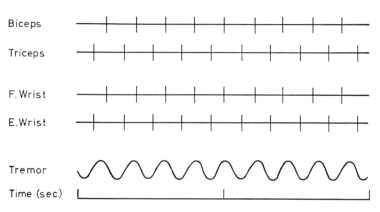

Biceps

Triceps

F. Wrist

E. Wrist

Tremor

Time (sec.)

98

must also be distinguished from 'intention tremor' which is a sign of cerebellar disease. Action tremor may be apparent in Parkinsonian patients at a stage of minimal rigidity, long before the more easily recognized alternating tremor emerges. An alternating tremor may never develop in some patients, but I have seen few unoperated

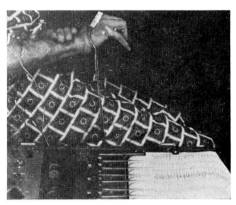

Figure 5.2. Action tremor in Parkinson's disease. The same patient as in Figure 5.1 is now flexing the elbow against the examiner's hand. The tremor, which is now an exaggerated physiological tremor, is synchronous in agonist and antagonist at 8–12 c/s

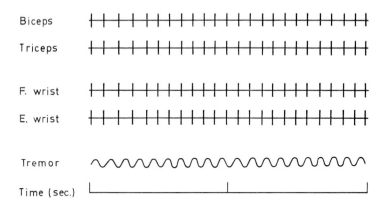

Biceps

Triceps

F. wrist

E. wrist

Tremor

Time (sec.)

patients with Parkinson's disease who did not have an action tremor. The differences between the action tremor and alternating tremor of Parkinson's disease may be summarized[18] as follows.

(1) The alternating tremor is so-called because the beats alternate between flexor and extensor groups, imparting a to-and-fro movement at a joint (*Figure 5.1*). A physiological tremor is a synchronous tremor (*Figure 5.2*). The beats appear simultaneously in agonist and antagonist so that the limb vibrates with a fine sinusoidal motion of

up to 1·2 mm in amplitude in normal subjects[31], increasing in Parkinson's disease and other conditions mentioned in the last section. It becomes clinically obvious as an action tremor.

(2) The frequency of alternating tremor is in the range 3–7 c/s and that of action tremor 7–12 c/s.

(3) Alternating tremor may be present at rest if the patient is in a state of nervous tension, but disappears if the patient is completely relaxed or asleep. It appears after a posture has been maintained for some time but usually ceases during voluntary activity whereas action tremor is a concomitant of muscular contraction.

One tremor mechanism is not a continuum of the other, that is, the alternating tremor does not gradually increase in frequency or suddenly double to become an action tremor. This would involve a change in character from alternating to synchronous tremor, as well as a change in frequency. Usually there is a distinct gap in EMG recordings between the cessation of one mechanism and the start of the other. It should be stated that there are some patients whose resting tremor is so gross that it may persist during activity with unaltered frequency and character and thus prevent the appearance of an action tremor.

Herringham[12], in 1890, noted both forms of tremor and commented 'in tranquil intervals patients with paralysis agitans have given natural effort tracings, with about 10 curves a second, but when shaking much the large waves obscure those of voluntary contraction'.

(4) Alternating tremor may be abolished by surgical destruction of the ventrolateral nucleus of the thalamus with the preservation of a marked action tremor.

Damage to the internal capsule (or upper motor neurone anywhere in its course) diminishes both forms of tremor.

THE MECHANISM OF PHYSIOLOGICAL TREMOR

Halliday and Redfearn[10] considered that physiological tremor was the result of an instability of the servo mechanisms of the stretch reflex arc, that is, an expression of the cycle of muscle contraction and relaxation which takes place because of the unloading of the muscle spindle during muscle contraction. There are a number of arguments against this. Clonus, which is caused by an exaggeration of this cycle in spasticity, is generally at about 7 c/s, a lower frequency than physiological tremor. Secondly, the frequency of physiological tremor is fairly constant in all parts of the body, irrespective of the length of the stretch reflex of the muscle concerned. Facial muscles may show physiological tremor at about 10 c/s, the same frequency as that

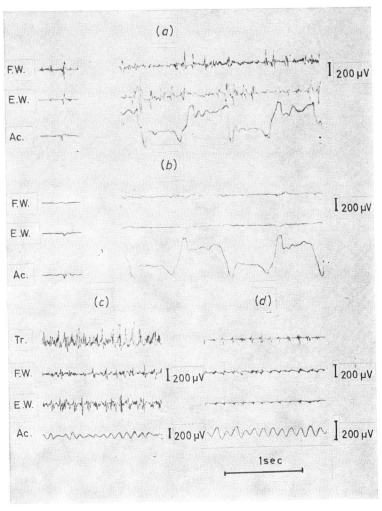

Figure 5.3. Persistence of exaggerated physiological tremor after ischaemic block of group Ia afferent fibres in a patient with Parkinson's disease. (a) Before the limb is rendered ischaemic, the radial jerk is recorded from the brachioradialis muscle in surface leads from flexors (F.W.) and extensors (E.W.) of the wrist. The characteristic pattern of cogwheel rigidity in stretched muscles is seen on the right, with the accelerometer tracing indicating passive movement of the wrist upwards and downwards; (b) after 32 minutes' ischaemia, the radial jerk and responses to passive movement are absent, indicating that the stretch reflex arc is blocked; (c) extension of elbow before ischaemia, showing exaggerated physiological tremor in triceps (Tr) and wrist muscles; (d) extension of elbow after 32 minutes' ischaemia, showing that the grouped action potentials of physiological tremor persist despite block of the stretch reflex arc (reproduced from Lance et al[18], by courtesy of the Editor of 'Brain')

recorded from the gastrocnemius[18, 24]. One would have to postulate that the shorter reflex arc of the facial muscles is compensated by a longer time for contraction of facial muscles, which seems most improbable, in order to account for a cycle of the same frequency. Thirdly, the mean position of the fingers with the hands outstretched fluctuates much more widely than the small rhythmic variations of physiological tremor, which argues against the tremor being caused by oscillations in a regulatory mechanism sensitive to displacement[31].

The fourth point, and one which seems conclusive, is that the stretch reflex arc may be interrupted by rendering the limb ischaemic, without altering the tremor rhythm recorded from contracting muscles (*Figure 5.3*). To support this, a physiological tremor has been demonstrated in a patient whose upper limb had been deafferented for intractable pain[23].

It is clear therefore that physiological tremor is determined by a central mechanism. The similarity in frequencies between physiological tremor and the alpha rhythm of the occipital cortex of the brain led investigators to correlate the two rhythms on the assumption that cortical rhythms might be propagated down descending motor pathways, but they have failed to show any link between cortical and tremor rhythms. Moreover, an action tremor of 10 c/s may be recorded during reflex withdrawal responses in patients below the level of a complete spinal section[24]. Buskirk and Fink[3] sought to relate physiological tremor to the ballistocardiogram, but since the tremor rhythm may be discerned in the EMG of contracting muscles, it must have its origin in neuromuscular activity and is not simply a movement artefact determined by the force of the heart beat.

The mechanism remains unknown but the most attractive postulate is that of central synchronization of motor neurone activity at about 10 impulses each second, whether motor neurones are thrown into tonic activity by descending motor pathways or by segmental reflex mechanisms. The central mechanism concerned is probably the recovery process of afferent terminals making synaptic contact with the motor neurone.

LESIONS OF THE LOWER MOTOR NEURONE

The alpha cell is the lower motor neurone. The alpha cell body lies in the anterior horn of the spinal cord grey matter, its dendrites receiving synaptic contacts directly from group Ia afferents and some descending motor tracts, as well as those from other reflex and motor pathways via internuncial cells. Alpha axons are of large diameter (maximum peak 15 μm) just a little smaller than group Ia afferents. Their fastest fibres have a mean conduction velocity of approximately 56 m/s in the upper limb and 50 m/s in the lower limb in man[32]. Alpha axons traverse the anterior root and usually a nerve root plexus (brachial or lumbosacral plexus), and mixed muscle nerve. Each axon is distributed to a number of muscle fibres which constitute a 'motor unit'. A lower motor neurone lesion leads to wasting and often fasciculation of the appropriate motor units.

All the motor axons in a muscle nerve may be stimulated electrically to produce a maximal muscle twitch, caused by simultaneous contraction of all motor units in the muscle. If the muscle is then stimulated reflexly, for example, by the H reflex in the case of the gastrocnemius-soleus complex in the calf, an estimate may be made of the amount of the motor neurone pool accessible to reflex activation. This varies from about 25 per cent to 100 per cent in different subjects. Any damage to the anterior horn cell motor pool will therefore be reflected by reduction in reflex activity proportionate to the diminution in voluntary activity. If the lower motor neurone lesion is associated with damage to afferent fibres as in peripheral neuropathy, the monosynaptic arc may be interrupted on the afferent side and tendon jerks may be lost before weakness is far advanced. Diminution or loss of reflexes is limited to the territory of the spinal cord segments or peripheral nerves affected.

Tonic stretch reflexes are also diminished or absent because of damage to the efferent limb of the monosynaptic arc. The resistance of the limb to passive movement at a joint is simply that of the elastic tension of ligaments and muscle, and the flail-like 'floppy' limb is said to be hypotonic. In the case of a normal subject who is able to relax completely a similar sensation of hypotonia may be felt by an examiner, because of voluntary cessation of both alpha and gamma cell activity so that no voluntary or reflex resistance to displacement can be elicited. Cerebellar damage may reduce gamma efferent discharge and thus tonic stretch reflex activity to a point where hypotonia is comparable with that of a lower motor neurone lesion. However, phasic muscle reflex activity is preserved in cerebellar lesions and tendon jerks remain active unlike the case of a lower motor neurone lesion.

Because of the hypotonic paralysis resulting from a lower motor neurone lesion, the affected limb assumes a posture determined not only by the mechanical structure of the limb and the force of gravity, but by the action of muscles whose nerve supply remains intact. The foot may thus acquire an appearance similar to that of pes cavus, which must be clearly distinguished from congenital pes cavus which

103

is usually hereditary, and frequently associated with other developmental anomalies in the nervous system.

It is an old warning, worth repeating, that a lesion of the lower motor neurone producing muscular paralysis which prevents flexion or extension of the great toe makes interpretation of the plantar response hazardous, since it may be possible for the toe only to flex or only to extend, whatever the nature of the reflex would have been in the intact limb. The physical signs of a lower motor neurone lesion are summarized in Table 5.1.

TABLE 5.1

Characteristics of Various Forms of Motor Disturbance

	LESION			
	lower motor neurone	*upper motor neurone*	*basal ganglia (Parkinsonism)*	*cerebellum*
Eventual posture	determined by distribution of weakness	flexed upper limbs; extended lower limbs	flexed upper and lower limbs	head held to side of lesion
Wasting	marked	slight	slight	none
Involuntary movements	fasciculation	flexor spasms	action tremor alternating tremor	intention tremor
Distribution of weakness	segmental or peripheral	extensors in upper limbs; flexors in lower limbs	none until late in the disease	none
Tonic stretch reflexes ('tone')	decreased	increased	increased	decreased
Phasic stretch reflexes ('tendon jerks')	diminished or absent	increased; clonus may be present	normal or slightly increased	normal or slightly increased
Co-ordination	impaired by weakness	impaired by weakness and spasticity	impaired by rigidity	specifically impaired (dysmetria, dysdiadochokinesia etc)

LESIONS OF THE UPPER MOTOR NEURONE

The upper motor neurone comprises the pyramidal tract and its associated extrapyramidal pathways. The pyramidal tract is rarely damaged in isolation, and it is known that an experimental lesion limited to the pyramidal tract does not produce frank spasticity. It is not possible to specify the exact way in which disease in the vicinity of the pyramidal tract augments muscle tone, but it is probable that the tract is shadowed in its course through the brain, brain-stem and spinal cord by fibres which normally exert an inhibitory effect upon the stretch reflex arc. These fibres arise from the motor cortex and the 'extrapyramidal cortex' anterior to the motor cortex and influence muscle tone through the inhibitory reticulospinal system (see Figures 4.5 and 4.6). The fibres must decussate at about the same level as the pyramidal tract, since the effect of a lesion in one lateral column of the spinal cord is strictly unilateral in man.

The normal function of upper motor neurone pathways in man is to interrupt the reflex standing (anti-gravity) pattern of muscle contraction in order to mediate voluntary movement. For this reason, disturbance of upper motor neurone function in man leads to a typical distribution of weakness since support is withdrawn from the extensor synergy in the upper limb and the flexor synergy in the lower limb. The distribution of weakness in the upper limbs involves abductors more than adductors, and extensors more than flexors. If the lesion is progressive, skilled movements of the distal muscles suffer before weakness may be detected in proximal muscles. In the lower limbs, the power of flexor groups is diminished before that of extensor groups. Since many antagonistic muscles derive part of their nerve supply from the same spinal segments, there is no way in which flexors and extensors can be afflicted differentially except by disorder of the upper motor neurone.

Although voluntary control of muscle is reduced or lost as a result of an upper motor neurone lesion, the muscles are still susceptible to reflex contraction because the lower motor neurone and many of its sources of reflex drive are still intact. For this reason, muscle wasting is slight compared with the gross changes of a lower motor neurone lesion. There is no fasciculation or fibrillation unless there has been secondary compression of peripheral nerves as a result of faulty posture. Some involuntary movements may take place as a result of reflex action, but these involve flexor or extensor synergies which have been released from supraspinal control.

Spasticity
Immediately following an upper motor neurone lesion, both extensor and flexor mechanisms are inert and it may take hours or days for reflex activity to become re-established. This quiescent period is known as the phase of cerebral or spinal 'shock'[13]. Extensor reflex mechanisms usually recover first in the lower limbs as under normal circumstances they are predominantly inhibited by the upper motor neurone. The lower limbs assume a posture of extension and any

105

attempt to flex the limb at a joint meets with resistance which increases in proportion to the velocity of stretch of extensor muscles. As stretch continues, the tonic stretch reflex is inhibited by the activity of Golgi tendon organs and secondary spindle endings and the

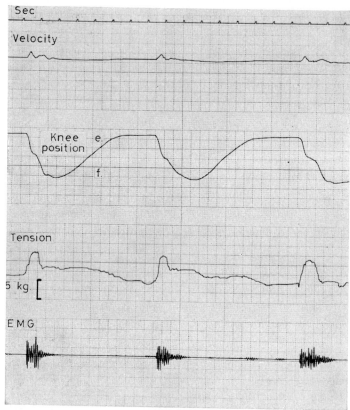

Figure 5.4. Spasticity. The patient is lying in the supine position with the leg being moved passively from a position of extension (E) to a position of flexion (F) at the knee joint. Tracings, from above downward, indicate velocity of displacement, angle of displacement at knee joint, force exerted at the ankle by the examiner's hand (as an indication of muscle tension) and EMG of quadriceps. It can be seen that passive flexion at the knee induces a tonic stretch reflex which increases, then disappears as flexion continues (clasp-knife effect). The clasp-knife effect is demonstrated in displacement and tension records as well as the EMG (from Burke, Gillies and Lance (1970). J. Neurol. Neurosurg. Psychiat., in the press)

stretched muscle suddenly relaxes—the 'clasp-knife' effect (*Figure 5.4*). The clasp-knife effect is not always obtained and some patients with upper motor neurone lesions show an increased resistance to passive stretch throughout the range of joint movements, which resembles that found in Parkinson's disease. The probable explanation for this is that inhibition mediated by group Ib and group II afferent fibres may be suppressed if the brain-stem is still in communication with the spinal cord[22]. In other patients with upper motor neurone lesions, increased resistance may be sensed only in the middle of the movement range with a critical muscle length and velocity of stretch. This is felt as a sudden slowing or 'catch' in the movement. Once the knee joint has been flexed beyond the clasp-knife point in a spastic patient, no tonic stretch reflex may be palpable, probably because of group II afferent inhibition and the knee jerk may even become pendular with the leg in the flexed position (Burke, Gillies and Lance, unpublished data).

Spasticity may be produced by ablation of the motor cortex in the monkey, but not by isolated section of the pyramidal tract in the medulla. In the early stage of spasticity the increase in tonic stretch reflexes is probably caused mainly by hyperactivity of the gamma efferent system so that blockade of the gamma efferent by procaine infiltration of muscle or muscle nerve or procaine infusion into the spinal canal, will abolish the tonic stretch reflexes. The intrathecal injection of phenol, which blocks small fibres preferentially like procaine, has been used to reduce stretch reflexes[26], although spasticity may return after several years. Dilute alcohol injected into muscle motor points will also reduce spasticity, probably by causing demyelination of the small fibres supplying the muscle spindle[11]. Landau and Clare[20] consider that there is no need to postulate increase in gamma efferent activity since H reflexes (which by-pass the muscle spindle mechanism) are augmented in hemiplegia. The significance of this is difficult to assess because the H reflex is potentiated by spindle afferent discharge.

In any case, after spasticity has been established for some time, there is a change in emphasis from gamma to alpha mechanisms. The upper limbs become fixed in flexion and the lower limbs tend to become fixed in extension, the dystonic posture. The posture of the upper limbs is influenced by the position of the head and neck if the brain-stem is still in contact with spinal centres. Denny-Brown[5] has shown that the dystonic state is not abolished by section of dorsal nerve roots, that is, it depends upon alpha motor neurone hyper-exitability, not upon the gamma loop.

When the upper motor neurone pathway is damaged in the spinal cord, imbalance between spinal inhibitory and facilitatory mechanisms, which were discussed in the previous chapter, results in spasticity. The tonic stretch reflex in spasticity is not only increased but is altered in character. It is of rapid onset and lacks the progressive augmentation of the normal response. It is best described as a stretch reflex which has been short-circuited in a state of facilitation, being deprived of normal supraspinal control. In spinal lesions, flexor and extensor mechanisms are enhanced and normal reciprocal innervation may be lost[6]. Flexor reflexes are initiated by visceral or cutaneous afferent impulses. Extensor reflexes may be overcome by flexor reflexes in the paraplegic patient when the bladder becomes distended or infected, or when nerve endings become distorted in the inflammatory oedema surrounding bed sores. The dominance of flexor reflexes is then manifested clinically by flexor spasms, and may finally result in a dystonic posture with the legs in a flexed position (paraplegia in flexion).

While tonic stretch reflexes are enhanced differentially in spasticity, phasic stretch reflexes are augmented in both flexors and extensors. All tendon jerks are hyperactive. The resumption of stretch after a reflex contraction is often sufficient to discharge muscle spindles again and produce another reflex contraction. The monosynaptic arc may thus be discharged repeatedly if stretch is maintained, a phenomenon known as clonus. The H reflex is increased in amplitude[20] and H reflexes may be recorded from many muscles where they were not apparent before. The recovery of the H reflex after a conditioning shock takes place more rapidly than in normal subjects[35]. The general enhancement of all phasic muscle reflexes leads to the phenomenon of reflex spread or irradiation, whereby a vibration wave propagated from a point of percussion is sufficient to trigger off 'tendon jerks' by stimulating the spindles of all muscles which lie in the path of the vibration wave. When spasticity is gross, the tendon jerks may be occluded as the tonic stretch reflexes occupy the whole motor neurone pool.

In distinction to deep muscle reflexes, superficial reflexes such as the corneal response, the superficial abdominal and cremasteric reflexes are diminished because they, being part of the flexor or protective reflex system, are normally facilitated by the intact upper motor neurone.

The extensor plantar response

One protective reflex which is altered completely in character by an upper motor neurone lesion is the plantar response, the clinical significance of which was first noted by Babinski. In normal mature man, stimulation of the sole of the foot results in a downward movement of the great toe. If the upper motor neurone has been damaged, stroking the lateral aspect of the sole will usually cause the great toe to extend. Since anatomical extension of the great toe is really a part of a physiological flexion reflex, the extensor plantar response may be regarded as a partial, uncontrolled protective flexion reflex[16]. In the infant, it may be seen as part of a generalized flexor withdrawal response in which the whole flexor synergy co-operates in removing the lower limb from an unpleasant stimulus to the sole of the foot. As the child becomes more mature and starts to stand and walk, flexor mechanisms fall more and more under the control of descending motor pathways, since they are used for many of the patterns of voluntary movement. The field from which the extensor plantar response may be elicited retracts until it consists only of the tip of the great toe. If the mature adult suffers damage to the upper motor neurone, the receptive field for the extensor response widens to include the whole of the first sacral dermatome on the sole and the lateral aspect of the foot. It is often useful to test the reflex by stroking the lateral aspect of the foot rather than the sole because it obviates the voluntary withdrawal of a ticklish patient which obscures the nature of the reflex response.

In a patient with complete destruction of the upper motor neurone in the spinal cord, there may be a flexor withdrawal response of the lower limb, and the receptive field often incorporates the greater part of the lower limb so that the response may be brought about by stimulation of any part of the calf or even of the thigh. The extensor plantar response may be termed an 'upgoing toe' or 'Babinski response'. The flexor plantar response may be termed a 'downgoing toe' but not a 'negative Babinski response' since it is the normal reflex in mature man. If the Babinski response has to be attributed to a lesion of a particular tract, it can be regarded as indicating a pyramidal disturbance, but it is more logically regarded as a spinal flexor reflex which is inadequately regulated because of defective upper motor neurone control. The plantar response is essentially a superficial reflex mediated through the first sacral segment and is therefore absent when sensory fibres supplying the sole and lateral aspect of the foot are damaged. The plantar response may become extensor during episodes of suppressed cortical activity such as hypoglycaemic or post-epileptic coma. It may remain flexor on occasions when all other signs point to an upper motor neurone lesion, so that an extensor plantar response must not be regarded as essential for the diagnosis of an upper motor neurone lesion. The physical signs generally encountered in upper motor neurone lesions are compared with those of other disorders in Table 5.1.

EXTRAPYRAMIDAL (PARKINSONIAN) RIGIDITY

Parkinson's disease and some other degenerative disorders of the basal ganglia are also associated with increased tonic stretch reflexes, which must be distinguished from the spasticity of upper motor neurone lesions.

There are a number of differences between extrapyramidal rigidity and upper motor neurone spasticity.

(1) Spasticity is commonly associated with weakness of extensors in the upper limb and flexors of the lower limb. Extrapyramidal rigidity is associated with weakness only in its advanced stages and even then it is difficult to determine whether muscle strength is diminished or simply impaired by muscle rigidity.

(2) The augmentation of tonic stretch reflexes is distributed differently in the two conditions. Flexors and extensors of the wrist are usually affected equally in Parkinson's disease whereas the flexors are more involved in spasticity. Dorsiflexors of the ankle are usually affected more than plantar flexors by rigidity whereas the reverse is the case in spasticity. Neck and trunk muscles are implicated more by rigidity. Facial muscles are affected equally in both disorders. Tonic stretch reflexes are increased in biceps brachii more than the triceps in both conditions and the quadriceps is affected more than the hamstrings in both, at least in the early stages. In advanced Parkinson's disease, all flexor groups become progressively more involved so that the patient adopts a dystonic posture in an attitude of flexion.

(3) Vibration-induced tonic contraction is normal in Parkinson's disease but is diminished or altered in character in patients with upper motor neurone lesions[17]. This suggests that normal supraspinal reflex pathways are intact in extrapyramidal rigidity but that function of the descending motor limb is impaired in spasticity. It is as though the Parkinsonian state is simply an exaggeration of normal mechanisms, which accounts for the pseudo-Parkinsonian cogwheel rigidity found in some anxious persons, whereas spasticity is the result of a short-circuit in the reflex pathway because of failure of spinal inhibition normally regulated from above.

(4) The dystonic attitude of advanced spasticity and rigidity involves flexion of the upper limbs. In Parkinson's disease the lower limbs also become flexed and the trunk may bow forward (flexion dystonia), while in upper motor neurone lesions, the lower limbs usually become fixed in extension with plantar flexion of the ankles (extension dystonia).

110

(5) The tonic stretch reflex of spasticity is usually interrupted at a certain degree of tension by the 'clasp-knife effect' (*Figure 5.4*). The tonic stretch reflex of extrapyramidal rigidity never builds up to this point but is interrupted at frequent intervals by the 'cogwheel effect'. The cogwheel effect is often sufficiently regular to be characterized as a rhythm in the range 4–14 c/s, and probably represents interruption of the tonic stretch reflex by the resting tremor or exaggerated physiological tremor of Parkinson's disease, whichever is engaging the motor neurone pool at the moment of testing (*Figure 5.5*).

(6) Tendon jerks are increased in spasticity but are usually within the normal range in Parkinson's disease. Upper motor neurone lesions augment both tonic and phasic stretch reflexes while Parkinson's disease usually enhances only tonic stretch reflexes. In contrast to both, cerebellar lesions usually diminish tonic stretch reflexes and yet may be associated with normal or increased phasic reflexes.

The fact that rigidity and spasticity both depend upon increased tonic stretch reflexes has been well shown by Rushworth[29]. Previously Matthews and Rushworth[25] had found that procaine blocked gamma efferent fibres before alpha fibres so that the application of procaine to a peripheral nerve or its injection into muscle provided a useful method of temporarily de-efferenting the muscle spindle while retaining virtually normal muscle power. It had long been known that procaine blocked small fibres before large, and its widespread use as a local anaesthetic relied upon its ability to block the small fibres which served pain sensibility differentially. It has recently been argued that procaine does block some afferent fibres of larger diameter at the same time as it abolishes conduction in small afferent and efferent fibres[7]. In spite of this, the clinical application of the method results in abolition of tendon jerks with preservation of power (particularly if muscle infiltration is used rather than perineural injection), so that it seems acceptable as a form of differential block. Using the technique of procaine infiltration of muscle, Walshe[33] had shown that Parkinsonian rigidity and spasticity could be reduced, and Rushworth[29] confirmed by EMG recordings that the increased tonic stretch reflexes of Parkinson's disease, as well as most cases of spasticity, could be selectively reduced by procaine nerve block (*Figure 5.6*). This indicates that hyperactivity of the gamma efferent system plays an important part in all these conditions although it is recognized that in some forms of spasticity and dystonia, the alpha motor neurones may be more active than the gamma system.

It would be an oversimplification to ascribe Parkinsonian rigidity solely to gamma hyperactivity. In normal subjects, as well as patients

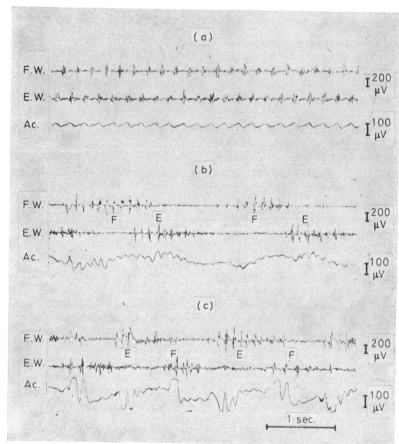

Figure 5.5. Parkinson's disease. The cogwheel phenomenon compared with alternating and physiological tremor in the same patient. (a) Alternating tremor at approximately 5 c/s. with the patient at rest; (b) Exaggerated physiological tremor at approximately 8 c/s. during voluntary movement (active flexion and extension of the wrist); (c) The cogwheel phenomenon appearing when flexors and extensors of the wrist are stretched alternately by passive movements of the wrist. The frequency of cogwheel beats is approximately 9 c/s., in the frequency range of physiological tremor. F. W. surface EMG from wrist flexors; E. W., surface EMG from wrist extensors; Ac., Accelerometer recording from hand; F., Flexion movement of wrist; E., Extension movement of wrist (Reproduced from Lance, Schwab and Peterson[18] by courtesy of the Editor of 'Brain')

with Parkinson's disease and spasticity, Landau, Weaver and Hornbein[19] obtained a clear differentiation between small and large fibre groups by inducing intrathecal or epidural block with procaine. Sensation to pinprick and temperature was lost while touch and proprioception remained intact. Tendon jerks were usually depressed 80 per cent or more before any muscle weakness became apparent in normal subjects. Diminution of rigidity, like that of spasticity, was closely related to the decrease of tendon jerks. Nevertheless, complete absence of spasticity and rigidity did not occur until there was significant loss of muscle strength. This observation has been confirmed[18] and suggests that the alpha cell is in a state of facilitation in both

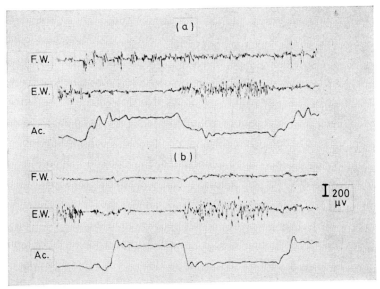

Figure 5.6. Abolition of Parkinsonian rigidity by infiltration of wrist flexors by procaine (a) Tonic stretch reflexes in wrist flexors and extensors. An upward deflection of the accelerometer tracing indicates that the wrist is being passively extended, and a downward deflection denotes passive flexion; (b) the stretch response is virtually abolished in wrist flexors after procaine infiltration of that muscle group, although power is unaffected, showing that gamma afferent fibres have been blocked by procaine (Reproduced from Lance, Schwab and Peterson[18] by courtesy of the Editor of 'Brain')

conditions and over-reacts to an afferent input which has been restored to normal levels. After a differential gamma efferent block by intrathecal procaine, Parkinsonian subjects may find it easier to move their limbs freely but suffer from a curious feeling of instability[15]. It is interesting that these patients do not show any 'cerebellar signs' although the afferent input to the cerebellum from the group Ia muscle spindle afferents must be grossly diminished.

When a patient is first seen with Parkinson's disease, suspicion may be aroused by the observation that the patient does not swing his arm freely on one or both sides. In the early stages of the disease, it may be difficult to confirm this suspicion by eliciting rigidity with passive movement of the patient's wrist, elbow or shoulder joints. It is helpful to get the patient to 'reinforce' by clenching a fist, turning the head from side to side or making a mental calculation. Cogwheel rigidity will then become apparent in a Parkinsonian patient.

The cogwheel phenomenon in Parkinson's disease

It seems reasonable to concede that the basis for both rigidity and spasticity is an increase in tonic stretch reflexes, and we must consider in more detail the possible explanation for the difference between the 'clasp-knife' and the 'cogwheel' phenomena. Certain reflexes between agonist and antagonist are exaggerated in Parkinson's disease. When the foot is suddenly dorsiflexed in Parkinsonian patients, the shortened muscles contract (Westphal phenomenon). This is due to proprioceptive discharge from antagonists and disappears when these are injected with procaine[30]. Its presence indicates that spinal segmental mechanisms are biassed towards alternating activity in agonist and antagonist, and therefore receptive to the superimposition of alternating tremor. The spinal mechanism of physiological tremor is also exaggerated in Parkinson's disease. If the two sides of a patient with unilateral disease are compared by means of EMG and accelerometer recordings, a normal physiological or action tremor will be found on the sound side, and a tremor of similar characteristics but much greater amplitude will be found on the side affected by other components of the Parkinsonian syndrome. This can be detected clinically as an action tremor in many patients who have no suggestion of a resting tremor.

The cogwheel effect lies more often in the frequency range of physiological (action) tremor than of resting tremor[18] but if resting tremor is predominant in a particular patient at a particular time then it will dictate the frequency of the cogwheel phenomenon (*Figure 5.7*). The alpha motor neurone is thus regulated by either resting or physiological tremor mechanism, whether it be discharged reflexly by group Ia afferents or driven from the pyramidal tract during voluntary movement. This appears to be a satisfactory hypothesis for the cogwheel effect, which could also explain why the clasp-knife phenomenon cannot be elicited in Parkinson's disease. Because the tonic stretch reflex is continually interrupted by tremor mechanisms, the muscle is unable to build up sufficient tension to evoke Golgi tendon organ discharge. Another factor, which may prove to be of greater importance, is the suppression of group Ib and group II reflex inhibition by the brain-stem. This inhibitory mechanism is intact in Parkinson's disease but is interrupted in most instances of spasticity.

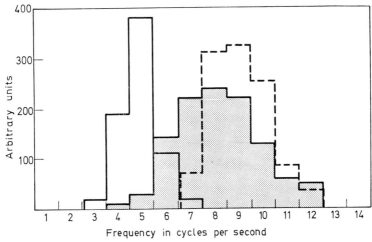

Figure 5.7. Graph illustrating the range of frequencies of alternating tremor (continuous line), physiological tremor (interrupted line) and the cogwheel phenomenon (shaded area) in 30 Parkinsonian patients, showing that the frequency of cogwheel rigidity is more often in the range of physiological tremor (Reproduced from Lance, Schwab and Peterson[18] by courtesy of the Editor of 'Brain')

Phasic stretch reflexes in Parkinson's disease

There is no satisfactory explanation why the tendon reflexes are not consistently increased in Parkinson's disease. It has been postulated that the relative inefficiency of the Jendrassik manoeuvre in reinforcing tendon reflexes in Parkinson's disease indicates underactivity of the gamma efferent system[14]. As mentioned earlier, it is doubtful whether the Jendrassik manoeuvre relies entirely on the gamma system for its effect, but in any event, reinforcement may become apparent in Parkinsonian patients as rigidity diminishes during the course of intrathecal procaine block[18]. This demonstrates that the mechanism is intact and suggests that reinforcement may not previously have been possible because the motor neurone pool was occupied with tonic mechanisms. Why this should be so when brisk (and reinforcible) tendon jerks are so commonly present in spasticity is difficult to say. Perhaps the answer may be found to lie in spinal internuncial systems which are normally under supraspinal control,

115

but which permit segmental mechanisms to become dominant when supraspinal control is impaired in spasticity.

A 'starter function' is said to be deficient in Parkinson's disease as there is often difficulty in initiating movement voluntarily. The patient may 'freeze' when attempting to walk, particularly when emotionally upset or when his attention is distracted by some minor obstacle in his path. This bradykinesia may be the result of bias away from phasic mechanisms in favour of tonic mechanisms. It may be abolished by operation on the globus pallidus or ventrolateral thalamus so that it must be explicable by some reversible physiological change.

The way in which operation of the motor system is altered in Parkinson's disease and other extrapyramidal disorders will be discussed further in the next chapter.

SUMMARY

The excitability of the alpha motor neurone depends upon its reception of impulses from the group Ia muscle afferent (excitatory), the group Ib muscle afferent from the Golgi tendon organ (inhibitory) and group II muscle afferent (inhibitory to extensors) as well as facilitatory and inhibitory impulses from contralateral reflex pathways, intersegmental reflexes, spinal cord internuncial cells and descending motor pathways. The firing rate of the alpha motor neurone is regulated by a feedback mechanism, the Renshaw cell, as well as by the recovery processes of the afferent fibres which impinge on the alpha cell.

Physiological tremor varies from 7 to 12 beats per second with synchronous contraction in agonist and antagonist, and is only present when muscle is contracting, so that it may be termed 'action tremor'. It is increased in certain physiological conditions and some clinical disorders, including Parkinson's disease, but its characteristics are completely different from those of the alternating tremor in Parkinson's disease.

Lesions of the lower motor neurone interrupt the stretch reflex arc so that tonic and phasic stretch reflexes are diminished or lost. Muscles are denervated in the distribution of either spinal cord segments or peripheral nerves, depending upon the site of the lesion, and the muscle undergoes wasting since it is deprived of reflex as well as voluntary activation.

Lesions of the upper motor neurone (comprising the pyramidal tract and its associated extrapyramidal pathways) leads to weakness of the extensor synergy in the upper limbs and the flexor synergy in the lower limbs. Fine movements of distal muscles are impaired. Tonic and phasic reflex mechanisms are usually increased after the initial phase of shock, because both alpha and gamma motor neurones are hyperactive. Tonic reflexes are most marked in flexors of upper limbs and extensors of lower limbs, but phasic reflexes are commonly enhanced in flexors and extensors alike. The plantar response usually becomes extensor because of partial release of control of flexor withdrawal mechanisms in the lower limb. Tonic stretch reflexes are often inhibited by group Ib and group II afferent fibres to give the 'clasp-knife' phenomenon. Muscles do not waste since they are still accessible to reflex discharge. In long-standing cases the patient may assume a dystonic posture because of the persistence of alpha hyperexcitability. The increased tonic stretch reflexes of spasticity are not simply an exaggeration of the normal response but are altered in character, being deprived of supraspinal regulation.

The rigidity of Parkinson's disease, like spasticity, depends upon alpha and gamma cell overaction, but resembles more closely an exaggeration of the normal stretch response. Rigidity lacks the clasp-knife effect of spasticity, probably because group Ib and group II inhibition is still under the control of the brain-stem and because the tonic stretch reflexes of Parkinson's disease are interrupted by either resting or physiological tremor to produce the 'cogwheel phenomenon', which prevents sufficient tension being built up in the muscle to provoke the Golgi tendon organ mechanism. Tendon jerks are not usually increased in Parkinson's disease. A flexed dystonic posture is common in the later stages of the disorder.

The phenomena of spasticity and extrapyramidal rigidity are explained and contrasted.

REFERENCES

[1] Adrian, E. D. and Bronk, D. W. (1929). 'The discharge of impulses in motor nerve fibres. Part II. The frequency of discharge in reflex and voluntary contraction.' *J. Physiol., Lond.* **67**, 119–151

[1] Alvord, E. C. and Fuortes, M. G. F. (1953). 'Reflex activity of extensor motor units following muscular afferent excitation.' *J. Physiol., Lond.* **122**, 302–321

[3] Buskirk, C. Van and Fink, R. A. (1962). 'Physiological tremor. An experimental study.' *Neurology, Minneap.* **12**, 361–370

[4] Denny-Brown, D. (1929). 'On the nature of postural reflexes.' *Proc. R. Soc.* **B104**, 252–301

[5] Denny-Brown, D. (1966). *The Cerebral Control of Movement.* Liverpool; University Press

117

6 Dimitrijević, M. R. and Nathan, P. W. (1967). 'Studies of spasticity in man. I. Some features of spasticity.' *Brain* **90**, 1–30

7 Gassel, M. M. and Diamantopoulos, E. (1964). 'The effect of procaine nerve block on neuromuscular reflex regulation in man. An appraisal of the role of the fusimotor system.' *Brain* **87**, 729–742

8 Granit, R., Haase, J. and Rutledge, L. T. (1960). 'Recurrent inhibition in relation to frequency of firing and limitation of discharge rate of extensor motoneurones.' *J. Physiol., Lond.* **154**, 308–328

9 Granit, R., Pascoe, J. E. and Steg, G. (1957). 'The behaviour of tonic α and γ motoneurones during stimulation of recurrent collaterals.' *J. Physiol., Lond.* **138**, 381–400

10 Halliday, A. M. and Redfearn, J. W. T. (1956). 'An analysis of the frequencies of finger tremor in healthy subjects.' *J. Physiol., Lond.* **134**, 600–611

11 Hariga, J., Tardieu, G., Tardieu, C. and Gagnard, L. (1966). 'Effets de l' application d'alcool dilué sur le nerf. Partie I. Confrontation de l'étude dynamographique et de l' étude histologique chez le chat décérébré.' *J. Neurol. Sci.* **3**, 284–299

12 Herringham, W. P. (1890). 'On muscular tremor.' *J. Physiol., Lond.* **11**, 478–485

13 Hunt, R. S., Meltzer, G. E. and Landau, W. M. (1963). 'Fusimotor function. Part I. Spinal shock of the cat and the monkey.' *Archs Neurol., Chicago* **9**, 120–126

14 Jung. R. and Hassler, R. (1960). In *American Physiological Society Handbook of Physiology*. Ed. by J. Field. Sect. 1, Vol. 2, p. 863. Baltimore; Williams and Wilkins

15 Kjellberg, R. N., Todd, D. P., Schwab, R. S., England, A. C., Lance, J. W. and Sweet, W. H. (1961). 'Gait improvement in Parkinsonian patients by gamma motor neurone suppression.' *Trans. Amer. neurol. Ass.* **86**, 126–130

16 Kugelberg, E. (1948). 'Demonstration of A and C fibre components in the Babinski plantar response and the pathological flexion reflex.' *Brain* **71**, 304–319

17 Lance, J. W., de Gail, P. and Neilson, P. D. (1966). 'Tonic and phasic spinal cord mechanisms in man.' *J. Neurol. Neurosurg. Psychiat.* **29**, 535–544

18 Lance, J. W., Schwab, R. S. and Peterson, E. A. (1963). 'Action tremor and the cogwheel phenomenon in Parkinson's disease.' *Brain* **86**, 95–110

19 Landau, W. M., Weaver, R. A. and Hornbein, T. F. (1960). 'Differential nerve block studies in normal subjects and in spasticity and rigidity.' *Archs Neurol., Chicago* **3**, 10–23

20 Landau, W. M. and Clare, M. H. (1964). 'Fusimotor function. Part VI. H reflex, tendon jerk and reinforcement in hemiplegia.' *Archs Neurol., Chicago* **10**, 128–134

21 Lippold, O. C. J., Redfearn, J. W. T. and Vučo, J. (1957). 'The rhythmical activity of groups of motor units in the voluntary contraction of muscle.' *J. Physiol., Lond.* **137**, 473–487

22 Lundberg, A. (1964). 'Supraspinal control of transmission in reflex paths to motor neurones and primary afferents.' *Prog. Brain. Res.* **12**, 197–221

[23] Marsden, C. D., Meadows, J. C., Lange, G. W. and Watson, R. S. (1968). 'Effects of deafferentation on human physiological tremor.' *Lancet* **2**, 700–702

[24] Marshall, J. and Walsh, E. (1956). 'Physiological tremor.' *J. Neurol. Neurosurg. Psychiat.* **19**, 260–267

[25] Matthews, P. B. C. and Rushworth, G. (1957). 'The selective effect of procaine on the stretch reflex and tendon jerk of soleus muscle when applied to its nerve.' *J. Physiol., Lond.* **135**, 245–262

[26] Nathan, P. W. (1959). 'Intrathecal phenol to relieve spasticity in paraplegia.' *Lancet* **2**, 1099–1105

[27] Preswick, G., Stewart, R. D. H., O'Hara, P. and Murray, I. P. C. (1966). 'The value of muscle twitch and Achilles reflex recordings in thyroid disorders.' *Med. J. Aust.* **1**, 473–477

[28] Redman, S. J. and Lampard, D. G. (1967). 'Monosynaptic stochastic stimulation of spinal motoneurones in the cat.' *Nature, Lond.* **216**, 921–922

[29] Rushworth, G. (1960). 'Spasticity and rigidity: An experimental study and review.' *J. Neurol. Neurosurg. Psychiat.* **23**, 99–118

[30] Rushworth, G. (1962). 'Muscle tone and the muscle spindle in clinical neurology.' In *Modern Trends in Neurology 3*, p. 36. Ed. by D. Williams. London; Butterworths

[31] Tabary, J. C., Tardieu, C. and Tardieu, G. (1965). 'Le tremblement postural chez le sujet normal. Étude du maintien de la position.' *J. Physiol., Paris* **57**, 313–324

[32] Thomas, P. K., Sears, T. A. and Gilliatt, R. W. (1959). 'The range of conduction velocity in normal motor nerve fibres to the small muscles of the hand and foot.' *J. Neurol. Neurosurg. Psychiat.* **22**, 175–181

[33] Walshe, F. M. R. (1924). 'Observations on the nature of the muscular rigidity of paralysis agitans, and on its relationship to tremor.' *Brain* **47**, 159–177

[34] Wilson, V. J., Talbot, W. H. and Diecke, F. P. J. (1960). 'Distribution of recurrent facilitation and inhibition in cat spinal cord.' *J. Neurophysiol.* **23**, 144–153

[35] Yap, C-B. (1967). 'Spinal segmental and long-loop reflexes on spinal motoneurone excitability in spasticity and rigidity.' *Brain* **90**, 887–896

6—The Basal Ganglia and their Disorders

It was pointed out earlier that animals such as the cat suffer only minor inconvenience from the section of one pyramidal tract, and there is evidence that quite extensive surgical lesions of the cerebral peduncle in man may leave good control of movement[5]. It is thus apparent that extrapyramidal tracts exert considerable control over movement as well as posture in man. It is justifiable to use the term extrapyramidal system since the tracts comprising it share an essential unity of function in spite of the bewildering number of connecting neurones which intervene between cortex and anterior horn cell.

THE EXTRAPYRAMIDAL MOTOR SYSTEM

The action of the extrapyramidal system on spinal motor neurones is expressed largely through reticulospinal pathways. The linkage between extrapyramidal cortex, basal ganglia and reticular formation is fairly well understood. The system may be regarded as a succession of relatively short neurones which descend from the cortex through relay nuclei, often as multiple paths in parallel, to influence reticulospinal, vestibulospinal and propriospinal tracts. At each relay the flow of onward impulses is regulated, often by neurones projecting upstream from areas such as the subthalamic nucleus, substantia nigra and midbrain reticular formation which provide a feedback control mechanism. There is also an important loop which passes from the cerebral cortex through the basal ganglia and back to the cortex which adjusts motor activity in cortifugal fibres, including the pyramidal tract.

Area 6 and the limbic region (and in all probability many other areas of cerebral cortex) project to the putamen and caudate nucleus[10]. Many efferent fibres from putamen and caudate proceed to the globus pallidus, from which two bundles, the ansa and fasciculus lenticularis, span the internal capsule to the thalamus anterior to the ventrolateral nucleus, where they probably relay with neurones which project back to the cortex anterior to the motor strip. This projection completes a cortico-cortical circuit through the basal ganglia which regulates voluntary cortical motor function by a process of graded inhibition which is considered to be of importance in the smooth control of movement (*Figure 6.1*).

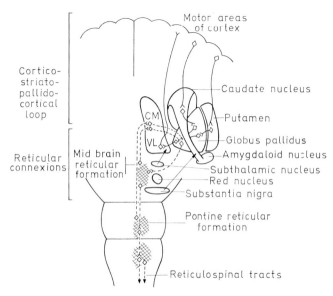

Figure 6.1. Connexions of the basal ganglia, simplified to illustrate the concept of two circuits concerned in the control of movement, linking the basal ganglia with the cortex and the midbrain reticular formation respectively. Arrows projecting rostrally from the subthalamic nucleus and substantia nigra denote that these nuclei exert a regulating or desynchronizing action on the above-mentioned circuits. CM, centrum medianum; VL, ventrolateral nucleus of thalamus (after Cooper[7])

As well as being part of the cortico-cortical feedback loop, the caudate nucleus and putamen receive fibres from the midbrain reticular formation via the centrum medianum of the thalamus[21] and project directly back to the midbrain reticular formation and the substantia nigra. This is a reciprocal relationship with the midbrain comparable with the cortico-striato-cortical connexions. Poirier and Sourkes have destroyed areas of the midbrain and pons in monkeys and subsequently estimated the catecholamine content of caudate nucleus and putamen. The concentration of dopamine and noradrenaline in these nuclei was found to be greatly reduced in those animals whose substantia nigra showed loss of cells. When the substantia nigra remained intact, the striatal catecholamine content was normal[37]. This provides valuable evidence of a nigrostriatal pathway.

The globus pallidus receives afferents from the ascending sensory tracts (medial lemniscus and spinothalamic tracts) and also fibres from the subthalamic nucleus and midbrain. As well as sending efferent fibres to the thalamus, the globus pallidus communicates with the subthalamic nucleus, the red nucleus and the adjacent midbrain reticular formation. It is probable that the fibres which project upstream from the midbrain reticular formation, substantia nigra and subthalamic nucleus to the basal ganglia have a regulatory effect upon motor function which is of clinical significance since damage to these structures is associated with involuntary movements.

The interstitial nucleus of the midbrain has been rather neglected by clinicians. It is responsible for rotational movements of the head and body. The interstitial nucleus has reciprocal connexions with the frontal eye movement fields (area 8), receives afferents from the vestibular nuclei and gives rise to an interstitiospinal tract which reaches down to the cervical cord[21]. It is a 'twist centre', part of the system for turning the head and rotating the body which may be implicated in the pathophysiology of organic torticollis and torsion spasm.

The extrapyramidal system is thus a democratic organization with a tenuous chain of command employing subcommittees which are constantly reporting back to a central committee, which in turn advises the board of directors. There is no need to question its traditional method as long as everything goes well, but its complexities make it difficult to determine the source of trouble if it ceases to function normally. It is unusual for a single symptom or sign to be correlated with a solitary lesion in the basal ganglia since degenerative changes are often widespread.

Certain facts may be observed from anatomical and physiological studies of experimental basal gangliar lesions or the ravages of disease which throw a subdued light on the nature of the neurological disturbance. It is certainly difficult to interpret the results of stimulation and ablation experiments in animals. Kennard[22] showed that no disability followed bilateral lesions of the caudate nucleus in monkeys unless cortical area 6 was removed simultaneously, in which case an 'action tremor' of 8–12 c/s appeared. Other authors have produced contralateral turning of the head and body, and sometimes circling movement by stimulation of the caudate nucleus. Extensive lesions in the monkey may be followed by running movements to the side of the lesion. Hodes, Peacock and Heath[19] showed that cortical motor activity could be suppressed by caudate stimulation, and it has been suggested that inhibition from the caudate nucleus is responsible for the interruption of the tonic phase of an epileptic seizure to produce the clonic phase[15]. Li[28] found that single shocks to the ventrolateral nucleus of thalamus arrested spontaneous activity in the motor cortex, and repetitive stimulation of this nucleus has been shown to depress responsiveness of corticospinal neurones to direct cortical stimulation[3, 4]. The cortico-caudato-thalamo-cortical loop thus appears to regulate the cortex through inhibition.

Gamma efferent activity is temporarily abolished by stimulation of the globus pallidus[19] and the ventrolateral nucleus of thalamus, providing the sensorimotor cortex is intact. If the effects of the gamma loop are eliminated by curarizing the animal, stimulation of these structures enhances the monosynaptic reflex by facilitating the alpha motor neurones[44]. Such facilitation again depends upon the sensorimotor cortex and is reversed or abolished by barbiturate anaesthesia. These experiments suggest that the basal ganglia are concerned with the balance of alpha and gamma mechanisms through their connexions with the motor cortex through the thalamus.

The substantia nigra is of particular interest because it projects rostrally to the caudate nucleus, putamen and probably globus pallidus, and because it degenerates in Parkinson's disease. Isolated destruction of the substantia nigra bilaterally in monkeys produces a tendency to immobility and slowness of movement without other Parkinsonian features[43], but if the dorsomedial part of the cerebral peduncle and an adjacent motor pathway descending from the region of the red nucleus (rubrotegmento-spinal tract) is interrupted as well in the monkey an alternating tremor develops on the opposite side of the body[38].

The ability of a monkey to return to the upright position after it has fallen depends on automatic adjustments (righting reflexes) requiring the integrity of the basal ganglia[10]. It is probable that afferent impulses resulting from body contact and position of the head travel from the spinal cord and the vestibular nuclei respectively to thalamus, and are then transmitted to globus pallidus, caudate and putamen. When these nuclei degenerate in man, abnormal postures result from imbalance of normal righting mechanisms.

The basal ganglia appear to be pecularly susceptible to anoxia, to paravascular degeneration and to the accumulation of substances such as copper (in Wilson's disease), calcium (in Fahr's disease or in hypoparathyroidism), bile pigments (in kernicterus) and iron (Hallervorden–Spatz disease), which indicates an unusual quality of the capillary network and the blood-brain barrier in this area[10].

PARKINSON'S DISEASE

James Parkinson, a general practitioner in Shoreditch, then a country village on the outskirts of London, published his monograph on *The Shaking Palsy* in 1817. He was a remarkable man. His published works include an authoritative book on fossils as well as a report of a case of appendicitis, and such treatises as *Dangerous Sports, Hints for the Improvement of Trusses* and *Observations on the Act for Regulating Madhouses*. He narrowly escaped being transported to Australia for his reformist activities. His life story[32] well repays reading. Parkinson's descriptions of the shaking palsy reads 'involuntary tremulous motion, with lessened muscular power, in parts not in action and even when supported; with a propensity to bend the trunk forwards, and to pass from a walking to a running pace: the senses and intellects being uninjured.'

Parkinson considered that the disease was one of the upper cervical cord and medulla. The centre of interest has now moved higher in the nervous system, but there is still no agreement about the precise localization of pathological change. Nor is this surprising, for a common feature observed in contrast radiography of the ventricular system (pneumoencephalography) in Parkinson's disease is the pooling of air in dilated cerebral sulci which indicates a diffuse atrophic process[42]. Pathological studies confirm the presence of generalized cerebral changes, which are essentially those of senility, with more severe lesions in the globus pallidus, substantia nigra and various brain-stem areas such as the dorsal motor nucleus of the vagus nerve. Cells in these areas are degenerated and frequently contain round hyaline bodies[17].

The symptoms of Parkinson's disease may appear in the third and fourth decade of life when the possibility of its being a sequel to encephalitis must be considered, although commonly no history of any illness resembling encephalitis can be elicited. Parkinson's disease and various dystonic phenomena, such as torticollis and oculogyric crises appeared in more than half the patients afflicted by encephalitis lethargica[12], and it is probable that post-encephalitic Parkinsonism still appears from time to time. The superimposition of dystonic postures on the pattern of Parkinson's disease suggests an encephalitic aetiology (*Figure 6.2*). Usually Parkinson's disease comes on in later life with or without associated signs of cerebral vascular disease. If vascular disease is present, there are usually signs of focal neurological damage elsewhere which may advance

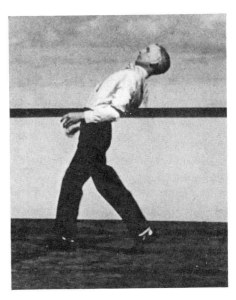

Figure 6.2. Dystonic posture assumed by a patient with Parkinson's disease on starting to walk. When standing still, posture was normal, although an alternating tremor of both upper limbs could be seen. (Patient photographed by courtesy of Dr. W. H. Wolfenden)

to bilateral disturbance of the upper motor neurone pathways above the brain-stem (pseudobulbar palsy). In this condition, areas of atherosclerotic softening or small cystic spaces can be demonstrated histologically in the basal ganglia and internal capsule. If there is no clinical indication of vascular disease, or past history of encephalitis, the condition is labelled 'idiopathic'. A family history of Parkinson's disease has been reported in 4 to 16 per cent of cases in different series[10]. The importance of upstream projections from midbrain to basal ganglia is emphasized by the fact that Parkinsonian tremor and rigidity may appear on one or both sides as the result of midbrain compression[35]. The signs of Parkinsonism may be found at various stages of Wilson's disease, and may appear transiently in hepatic encephalopathy or permanently in chronic liver disease irrespective of the cause. The syndrome may appear after carbon monoxide or manganese poisoning, and I have seen it after methyl bromide poisoning. It may appear reversibly or even permanently after the use of phenothiazine drugs such as chlorpromazine, or the use of reserpine.

Ehringer and Hornykiewicz[14] reported that the concentration of dopamine was reduced in the basal ganglia of Parkinsonian patients and it is now known that striatal dopamine content decreases substantially in monkeys after the substantia nigra is destroyed[37]. This leads to the attractive hypothesis that degeneration of the substantia nigra in Parkinson's disease is responsible for the loss of a dopaminergic nigrostriatal tract which normally controls striatal mechanisms. Dopamine inhibits the stretch receptor neurone of the crayfish[31] and has been considered as a possible inhibitory transmitter substance in man. Barbeau[2] stated that the excretion products of dopamine and serotonin are diminished in the urine in this disease but this is still open to question[36]. Barbeau postulated a block in the pathway of noradrenaline and serotonin formation as the result of defective action of the enzyme dopa decarboxylase. Reserpine causes discharge of noradrenaline and serotonin from body stores and would therefore deplete the basal ganglia of these amines, which could account for its action in producing or augmenting the signs of Parkinson's disease. Depression, which is usually a concomitant of Parkinson's disease, may also be related to depletion of cerebral amines. Alpha-methyl-dopa is known to worsen the tremor and rigidity of Parkinsonian patients and to produce these symptoms in subjects with a previously normal motor system. On the other hand, administration of L-dopa (3-16 g daily) decreases rigidity at the lower dosage levels and improves or abolishes tremor in higher doses[9].

The ability of the Parkinsonian patient to metabolize infused 5-hydroxytryptophane has been tested by measuring the urinary excretion of its derivatives, 5-hydroxytryptamine (5HT) and 5 hydroxy-indoleacetic acid (5HIAA)[40]. No difference was found between Parkinsonian patients and those with other neurological diseases and there was no amelioration of the tremor or rigidity by the infusion. Since only about 1 per cent of body 5HT is contained in the brain and the vast bulk (95 per cent) is in the gastro-intestinal tract, it is unlikely that any localized cerebral disturbance would be reflected in general metabolic studies.

The nature of the disturbance in Parkinson's disease
Parkinson's disease commonly presents with difficulty in using one arm for skilled movement, dragging one foot when walking, or the

complaint of aching in the affected limbs. The arm may not swing freely on walking and careful examination will disclose the presence of cogwheel rigidity on the affected side, particularly if the patient reinforces spinal mechanisms by turning the head from side to side or some similar motion. At this early stage, an increase in physiological tremor during firm muscle contraction (action tremor) can usually be demonstrated[24]. Sometimes alternating tremor may be the presenting sign, and it appears in most patients at some stage of the illness. If alternating tremor becomes so gross that it persists during muscular activity, it obliterates the action tremor. Excessive salivation and other autonomic disturbances are common[13], presumably related to degeneration of autonomic nuclei in the brainstem. Urgency of micturition with uninhibited bladder function has been noted in about 25 per cent of patients[33] suggesting that the basal ganglia may play a part in the control of bladder function. It is interesting in this connexion that stimulation of the globus pallidus inhibits spontaneous bladder contraction in the cat[27].

The nature of the disturbance of spinal cord mechanisms responsible for rigidity, action tremor and the cogwheel effect, has been discussed in earlier chapters. The exact way in which the balance of reticulospinal activity is altered so as to increase the tonic activity of both gamma and alpha motor neurones is unknown. It is possible that degeneration of the nigrostriatal tract alters the outflow from striatum and pallidum to the ventrolateral thalamus which in turn impairs the restraining effect of the frontal cortex upon muscle tone. The effect of basal ganglia degeneration on the reticular formation could be more direct than this, but it is difficult to see why surgical destruction of the ventrolateral thalamus should be as effective as destruction of the globus pallidus if the pallido-thalamo-cortical pathway is not involved in the production of rigidity. Parkinson's disease may thus be considered as the result of an unhibited frontal cortex with increased forebrain drive of spinal segmental mechanisms[25].

Hassler considered that the appearance of resting tremor resulted from reduction of activity of strio-nigro-reticular connexions which have a desynchronizing influence, so that the pallido-reticular tract is able to exert an unopposed synchronizing influence[21]. However, it seems more probable that the resting tremor of Parkinson's disease is generated in the cortico-strio-pallido-thalamo-cortical circuit. Experimental postural tremor in the monkey which resembles the alternating tremor of Parkinson's disease, is associated with loss of serotonin as well as dopamine from the striatum[38]. Pallidal or thalamic stimulation may produce the characteristic tremor in patients with Parkinson's disease but not in those patients with other movement disorders[47]. Discharges have been recorded from the thalamus of Parkinsonian patients at the same frequency as their tremor. It is probable that these thalamic rhythms were secondary to the tremor in some areas such as the main somatic sensory nucleus (ventralis posterior lateralis, VPL) and that the discharge in this case is derived from the activation of proprioceptors by the tremor. In other areas, such as lateralis posterior and the ventrolateral nucleus, the thalamic rhythms preceded tremor in the limbs and sometimes appeared in the absence of tremor[1, 18]. It is therefore possible that this thalamic activity could be related to the generation of tremor. Tremor, like rigidity, is abolished by a surgical lesion in globus pallidus or ventrolateral thalamus[7]. The tremor rhythm appears to be propagated from the cortex to the spinal cord along the pyramidal tract since interruption of the tract at any point abolishes the tremor[7, 34] but proof of this hypothesis must await the recording of a tremor rhythm from the tract. Bursts of impulses traversing the pyramidal tract could easily be transformed into an alternating tremor by the reciprocal innervation of segmental motor pathways. Pyramidal tract activity would tend to become desynchronized during voluntary activity and thus explain the disappearance of resting tremor during movement. When resting tremor ceases to dominate the anterior horn cell, the purely spinal mechanism of action tremor is able to do so.

It is probable that the connexions of the basal ganglia which are hyperactive in Parkinson's disease contain cholinergic synapses because anticholinergic substances are beneficial in their effects upon both tremor and rigidity. Phenothiazine derivatives and reserpine on the other hand increase rigidity. Purdon Martin[30] points out that postural fixation and righting reactions are impaired in advanced Parkinson's disease, which is to be expected since righting reactions are mediated through the basal ganglia and associated reticular formation.

HEMIBALLISMUS

This condition is one of the most dramatic of the dyskinesias. A patient suffering a thrombosis in the region of the subthalamic nucleus, or between that nucleus and the thalamus or pallidum, suddenly develops a wild swinging movement of the arm and leg on the opposite side of the body (*Figure 6.3*). One patient of mine awakened from sleep thinking that he was being attacked because he felt a succession of blows to one side of his body. He was startled to find that his own arm and leg were undergoing rotatory movements at shoulder and hip joint so that he was being hit by the flailing arm and leg on that side.

Hemiballismus may be regarded as a disorder of fixation of the proximal muscles of a limb which is necessary for the normal use of a limb[29]. It is of interest that a patient with the wild movements of hemiballismus may be able to fix the position of one hand for a period long enough to raise a glass to the lips and drink from it by making compensatory movements of the trunk muscles.

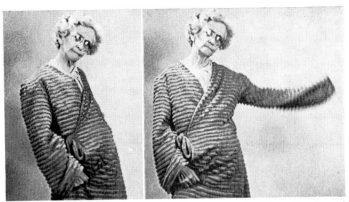

Figure 6.3. Hemiballismus. Frames from a cine film illustrating the wild swinging movements of the left upper limb with rotation of the trunk. (Patient photographed by courtesy of Sir Kenneth Noad)

It is probable that projections from the subthalamic nucleus rostrally to the thalamus and pallidum exert a steadying influence upon the outflow from the pallidum in the maintenance of posture. The movements of hemiballismus are such as would be expected from repetitive firing of extrapyramidal pathways, affecting tonic mechanisms sequentially so that a stereotyped movement is produced. Hemiballismus is the only involuntary movement which may continue during sleep and hence is presumably independent of the reticulo-spinal pathways. This is supported by the findings of Carpenter, Strominger and Weiss[6] that lesions of the centromedian and other intralaminar nuclei did not benefit experimental subthalamic dyskinesia in monkeys. Hemiballismus is suppressed by large doses of chlorpromazine, and has been abolished by operations upon the globus pallidus or ventrolateral nucleus of thalamus.

Hemiballismus tends to improve with time and if patients are observed as improvement occurs it will be seen that proximal muscles become less involved and that the residual movements seen in distal parts of the limb may bear a striking resemblance to those of chorea.

CHOREA

The term chorea is used to describe involuntary twitching of the face and limbs, affecting distal muscles as much as proximal. In EMG recordings, the muscle potentials resemble those of normal contraction except that the amplitude of the 'interference pattern' waxes and wanes and antagonistic muscles may be in action at inappropriate times[20]. While the movements are shorter in duration that those of athetosis, they are much longer than the shock-like contraction

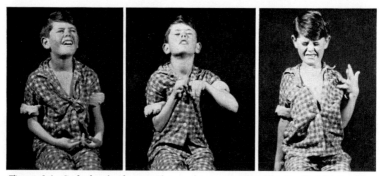

Figure 6.4. Sydenham's chorea. Frames from a cine film showing facial grimacing, involuntary movements on attempting to do up a button, and athetoid posturing

commonly seen in myoclonus (which stands out in the EMG as a synchronous spike resembling that of the tendon jerk). The disturbance in chorea is one of tonic rather than phasic mechanisms, but it differs from athetosis not only in the shorter duration of involuntary movement but in the failure to produce alternating or sustained postural changes. However it is often necessary to use the term 'choreoathetosis' in many patients, where movements of both types are present. Many children with transient rheumatic (Sydenham's) chorea or adults with progressive Huntington's chorea may have classical athetotic movements (*Figure 6.4*).

The pathological changes of Huntington's chorea are well known, but by the time the patient dies of this disorder, the nature has usually changed to that of a progressive dystonia with fixed abnormal posture and few involuntary movements. The neuronal degeneration in the frontal cortex and caudate nucleus is the most striking change, but putamen and cerebellum are also involved[17]. The pathology of rheumatic chorea is less well documented since the patient usually recovers spontaneously and completely. Cellular infiltration has been reported in cortex, basal ganglia and cerebellum; endarteritis may be present.

The clinical picture of rheumatic chorea is commonly that of a cerebellar syndrome affecting the limbs with or without ataxia of gait, in addition to involuntary facial contortions and twitching and writhing movements of the limbs. When the choreic patient is completely at rest, there may be little involuntary movement. When the patient walks, the hands may undergo extension movements at the fingers or wrists. This gives rise to an odd effeminate gesture of the hand which is often conspicuous as the patient turns while walking. The tongue may snap back after being protruded. A sustained grasp is not possible and continued variation in the grip is felt by the examiner. The abnormal movements are brought out by maintaining a posture or attempts at co-ordinated movement (*Figure 6.4*). Choreoathetotic movements become much worse as the goal is approached in the manner of intention tremor. This feature is so constant that it brings to mind the possibility of abnormal synchronization and repetitive neuronal firing in the cerebello-thalamo-cortical pathways as being part of the disturbed physiology in chorea.

Tonic stretch reflexes are commonly diminished in rheumatic chorea, as they are in most forms of cerebellar disease, whereas phasic reflexes are usually unaffected. This gives rise to the pendular knee jerk, which may have a secondary quadriceps contraction superimposed upon the reflex contraction to give the appearance of a sustained or 'hung-up' knee jerk (*Figure 6.5*).

Over a period varying from one week to two years rheumatic chorea usually resolves spontaneously[26]. In contrast, Huntington's chorea becomes progressively worse with the appearance of rigidity until eventually the patient assumes a dystonic posture with flexed upper limbs and extended lower limbs[10]. Uncommonly, patients with a family history of Huntington's chorea may suffer an illness of increasing rigidity terminating in dystonia, without ever showing involuntary movements.

Choreiform movements may be seen occasionally in atherosclerotic or senile brain disease, as the sequel to hypoxia, and as a symptom of uraemic, hepatic or hypercapnic encephalopathy. Choreo-athetoid movements were described by Poirier, Sourkes and their colleagues[38] as a transient abnormality after interruption of the nigro-striatal tract in the monkey. In two animals with sparing of the substantia nigra but destruction of the dorsomedial part of the cerebral peduncle and adjacent rubro-tegmento-spinal tract, choreiform and ballistic movements continued on the opposite side. Similar movements may occur in man after placement of a stereotactic lesion deeper than usual in the treatment of Parkinson's disease[39].

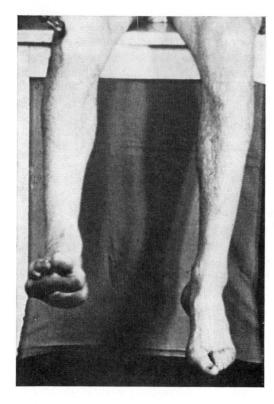

Figure 6.5. A 'Hung-up' knee jerk in Huntington's chorea. A choreic contraction of the quadriceps following the knee jerk is responsible for maintaining the leg in partial extension

The movements of Huntington's chorea can usually be controlled by the use of chlorpromazine in large doses such as 300–600 mg daily. No treatment may be necessary in rheumatic chorea, but diazepam (Valium) is helpful in reducing the involuntary movements as an alternative to phenothiazine derivatives.

ATHETOSIS

The movements of athetosis are slower than those classified as chorea and are exaggerated by voluntary movement.

Attempts at voluntary movement lead to a succession of abnormal postures, because of alternating adduction and abduction at the shoulder joint and flexion and extension at distal joints. Commonly, the wrist is flexed, but fingers are extended. The hand may approach an object, but be unable to grasp it because of the constant fluctuations in tonic contraction of postural muscles. The more severe the disorder, the greater is the tendency for flexion responses to predominate in the upper limbs and extension reactions in the lower limbs. Tonic stretch reflexes in the relaxed patient may be normal or diminished at first, but eventually resistance to passive movement becomes increased and the upper limbs may become fixed in flexion, and the lower limbs in extension (*See Figure 4.1*). This terminal dystonic posture is called the 'striatal position' because of its association with degeneration of the striatum, particularly the putamen[10]. Athetosis often coexists with choreiform movements (choreoathetosis) when muscle tone may be diminished, or with dystonia, in which case tonic stretch reflexes are enhanced, or with an upper motor neurone lesion, when both tonic and phasic stretch reflexes are increased.

Athetosis is usually the result of anoxia at the time of birth, but has been reported as part of the syndrome of post-anoxic encephalopathy in adults. It may be the result of encephalitis, usually in early childhood, or may appear as part of the symptom complex of kernicterus, Wilson's disease or other basal gangliar disturbances.

Tardieu and Tabary[46] point out that athetosis is peculiarly a reaction of childhood and is rarely seen in the brain-damaged adult. They postulate that the infantile brain has the ability to employ a variety of motor pathways in an attempt to replace those destroyed by disease.

The pathological changes in athetosis affect the putamen more than caudate nucleus, and cortical changes have been reported. Degeneration of nerve cells and gliosis frequently coexist with overgrowth of axis cylinders, which may represent an attempt at neural regeneration, and gives a marbled appearance to the corpus striatum.

Denny-Brown has shown that medial frontal lobe lesions release grasping and groping reactions, and lesions of the lateral aspect of the parietal lobe may lead to a withdrawal response with extension of the fingers—the 'avoiding reaction'. These reactions may be elicited in a patient with athetosis, and the grasp component is usually particularly striking. The movements of an athetotic patient suggest a sequence of grasp and avoiding reactions, and it is probable that the normal cortical control of these reflexes is mediated through

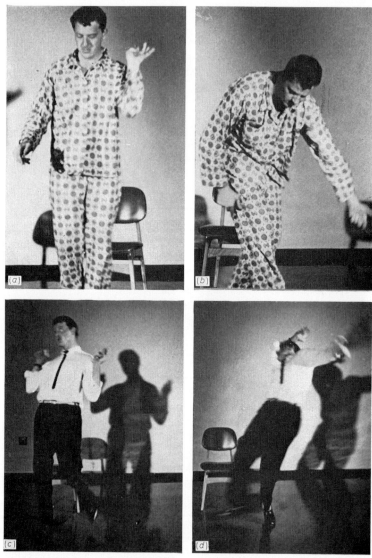

Figure 6.6. Paroxysmal choreoathetosis. Seizures precipitated by movement in which athetoid posturing (a) may be followed by ballistic movements of the limbs (b), which may become sufficiently violent to throw the patient to the ground (c, d) (Patient photographed by courtesy of Dr. R. D. Fine)

corticostriatal fibres so that they are released in athetosis when the relay station of their controlling fibres is damaged in the putamen[10]. Cortical control of the basal ganglia may be released transiently in the curious condition of paroxysmal choreoathetosis (*Figure 6.6*) in which episodes are triggered by attempts at involuntary movement and may be of sufficient violence to throw the patient to the ground[15].

DYSTONIA

Dystonia is a condition in which attempted voluntary movement leads to tonic contraction of antagonistic muscle groups so that part or whole of the body assumes an abnormal posture. Dystonia

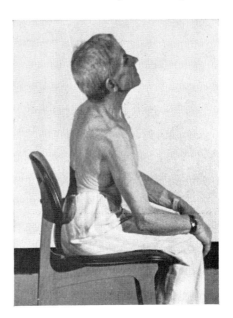

Figure 6.7. Retrocollis. The forced posture was accompanied by rhythmic jerking of the neck muscles, which was eased by bending forwards

may affect one part of the body only, such as the upper quadrant in writer's cramp, the neck musculature in spasmodic torticollis or retrocollis (*Figure 6.7*), or one leg in early dystonia musculorum deformans. Writer's cramp and torticollis may remain throughout life, fluctuating in intensity, without other signs of dystonia becoming apparent or they may be part of a general dystonic syndrome. Dystonia musculorum deformans extends to involve upper as well as lower limbs, often more on one side of the body than the other, in addition to the trunk muscles so that 'torsion spasm' of the body appears on standing and walking (*Figure 6.8*).   Posture tends to become fixed later in the disease with kyphoscoliosis, flexed upper limbs and extended lower limbs.   Dystonia musculorum deformans is an uncommon disease, appearing in childhood or adolescence. The usual pathological change in dystonia musculorum deformans is a marbled appearance of putamen and of thalamus which resembles closely that of double athetosis.   It is possible that such changes are initiated in childhood by a combination of fever and anoxia[10] and that a progressive gliosis commences at that time.

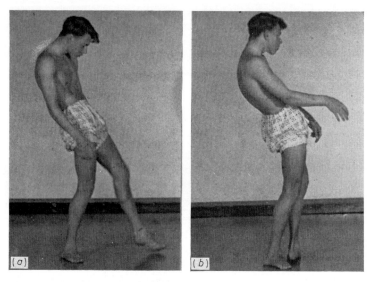

Figure 6.8.   Dystonia musculorum deformans.   On attempted movement agonistic and antagonistic muscles contract together, tending to fix the limbs (or trunk) in an abnormal posture

Dystonic manifestations are common in the later stages of most diseases of the basal ganglia.   Denny-Brown has described two basic dystonic postures recognized in advanced motor system disorders.   The flexed dystonic posture, in which both upper and lower limbs are flexed, is known as the 'pallidal position' and is seen after bilateral damage to the globus pallidus (for instance, in carbon monoxide poisoning) or in late Parkinson's disease.   The more common attitude of flexed upper limbs and extended lower limbs, known as the 'striatal position' may be seen as the end-result of a unilateral upper motor neurone lesion (for example, the 'contracture' of hemiplegia), or bilateral atherosclerotic disease of the putamen ('pseudobulbar palsy'), progressive choreoathetosis from birth anoxia, Huntington's chorea, Wilson's disease, post-encephalitic states or dystonia musculorum deformans.

Although the pathological changes of all these various disorders show an emphasis on different nuclei of the basal ganglia, those which end in the 'striatal position' all have degenerative changes involving the putamen. Progressive striatal lesions are responsible for increasing domination of posture by body-contact and labyrinthine righting reflexes. Denny-Brown considers that localized or 'segmental' dystonias such as spasmodic torticollis may result from selective damage to certain fibres entering the putamen.

Both flexion and extension dystonia have been produced by cortical ablation in the monkey[11]. Dystonia in the 'striatal' or hemiplegic posture follows bilateral removal of the parietal lobes and areas 6 and 8, which leaves the motor strip (area 4) isolated. Section of both eighth nerves removes labyrinthine influences on posture and leaves body-contact reflexes unopposed, which converts the hemiplegic posture to one of flexion of all four limbs. Such dystonic postures are mediated chiefly through hyperexcitability of alpha motor neurones. Gamma efferent activity is also increased in dystonia but affects flexor and extensor muscles equally, unlike the differential changes in spasticity[16].

Dystonia may be relieved by a variety of surgical lesions, more effective if bilateral. After analysis of operations on 130 cases of dystonia musculorum deformans, Cooper[8] has concluded that the lesion of choice is bilateral destruction of ventrolateral nucleus of thalamus, the anterior part of the specific sensory relay nuclei (postero-ventrolateral and postero-ventro-medial nuclei) and centrum medianum. Rand and Markham[39] reported favourably on the destruction of substantia nigra in addition to thalamic and pallidal lesions.

Possibly the most spectacular of iatrogenic diseases is the induction of dystonic symptoms by phenothiazine derivatives. Chlorpromazine will predictably induce Parkinsonian symptoms if the dosage is sufficiently high and in some cases a choreoathetotic syndrome has followed prolonged use of phenothiazine drugs, which has persisted after cessation of the treatment. One has seen many patients with trismus, asymmetrical spasms of tongue, face and jaw and the assumption of abnormal postures including opisthotonus, following the use of small doses of prochlorperazine, trifluoperazine, thiethylperazine and fluphenazine. A dramatic instance of such postural changes is shown in *Figure 6.9* by courtesy of Dr. G. Preswick, who was standing by with a Polaroid camera as the patient was admitted to hospital. The mechanism of transient drug-induced dystonia is unknown, but fortunately, it can be relieved immediately by the intravenous injection of benztropine methanesulphonate (Cogentin) 1–2 mg.

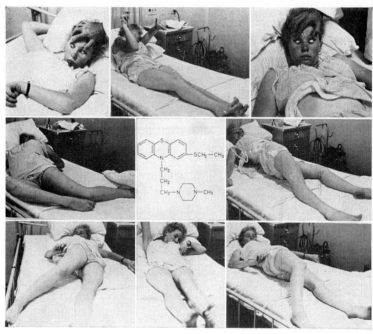

Figure 6.9.   Drug-induced dystonic seizures, which followed the ingestion of thiethylperazine, and were relieved promptly by benztropine methanesulphonate (Photographs by courtesy of Dr. G. Preswick)

Transient dystonic postures have been recorded as an apparently epileptic phenomenon, superimposed on extrapyramidal disorders, such as Wilson's disease, or choreoathetosis resulting from birth trauma or encephalitis. They may be symptomatic of a paracentral cortical lesion or of multiple sclerosis[23]. Such spasms may also occur in hypocalcaemia, or in otherwise healthy people as a reaction to being startled. The seizure is commonly unilateral, involving flexion of one arm and extension of the leg on the same side, the abnormal posture lasting only a few seconds or perhaps minutes, and may be precipitated by movement. The condition is called extrapyramidal or striatal epilepsy in the older literature, but is probably best described as dystonic seizures until the mechanism is clarified. The disorder is probably related to paroxysmal choreoathetosis, which was described earlier in this chapter and which is also precipitated by movement. Both must be distinguished from a familial tendency to prolonged dystonic posturing and involuntary movements, lasting from several minutes to several hours, which is precipitated by fatigue, excitement or alcohol rather than movement and has been

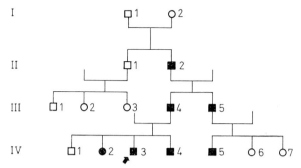

Figure 6.10. Paroxysmal dystonic choreoathetosis. Three generations of a family subject to dystonic seizures, which lasted 5–60 minutes on each occasion[23]. *The patient marked with the arrow has developed bouts of choreoathetosis, which indicates that this familial condition is a variant of paroxysmal dystonic choreoathetosis*[41]

called paroxysmal dystonic choreoathetosis[41]. In 1963, I reported a family in which members of three generations suffered from prolonged dystonic seizures[23], and I have recently seen a member of the family who was unaffected at that time, but has since developed episodic choreoathetosis which may last for hours at a time. This patient clearly establishes a link between the familial occurrence of dystonic seizures and paroxysmal dystonic choreoathetosis (*Figure 6.10*). The condition was presumably the result of a temporary failure of cortical control of basal gangliar mechanisms, the cause of which is unknown.

SUMMARY

The basal ganglia have important reciprocal connexions with both the cerebral cortex and midbrain reticular formation, and receive afferent fibres from the ascending sensory pathways via the thalamus. These connexions play an important part in righting reflexes, grasping and avoiding reactions, and the regulation of tone, posture and movement.

The extrapyramidal cortex projects through the neostriatum (caudate nucleus and putamen) and globus pallidus to the thalamus which then sends fibres back to the motor cortex. This cortico-striato-pallido-thalamo-cortical circuit exerts a restraining effect upon the motor cortex and area 6 anterior to it. Degeneration of the basal ganglia in Parkinson's disease permits rhythmic synchronous activity in this circuit which may be propagated down the pyramidal tract during periods of inactivity to produce an alternating tremor through reciprocal spinal cord mechanisms.

The neostriatum and globus pallidus are closely connected with the midbrain reticular formation and may thereby influence muscle tone more directly than via their cortical connexions. It is probable that ascending fibres from the substantia nigra, subthalamic nucleus and reticular formation have a regulatory effect upon the motor system, since lesions in this area release involuntary movements if there is co-existing damage in other parts of the midbrain or basal ganglia. The interstitial nucleus and its cortical, vestibular and spinal connexions mediate rotation of the head and body, and may be implicated in the production of torticollis.

Parkinson's disease is a degenerative disorder, the main brunt of which falls upon the basal ganglia, chiefly the substantia nigra. Striatal dopamine content is decreased, possibly as a result of degeneration in an inhibitory nigrostriatal pathway. The condition is characterized by increased tonic stretch reflexes, but not phasic reflexes, and both resting (alternating) and action tremors which interrupt the tonic stretch reflex, thus giving rise to 'cogwheel rigidity'. During periods of voluntary motor activity the alternating tremor is usually suppressed and an exaggerated physiological tremor (action tremor) is seen. Autonomic control of salivation and other gastrointestinal activity, and bladder function, may be impaired.

The mechanism of the dyskinesias such as hemiballismus, chorea and athetosis is not well understood. The involuntary movements of hemiballismus comprise a sequential activation of postural muscles which continues day and night. Chorea and athetosis, on the other hand, are initiated by maintaining posture or attempting voluntary movement. Athetosis has been explained by Denny-Brown as an alternation of grasp and avoiding reactions released by degeneration of cortico-striatal fibres which normally mediate these reactions through the putamen.

Dystonia is a condition in which antagonistic muscle groups contract together, tending to fix a part of the body in an abnormal posture. It is seen as the end result of many different disorders affecting the basal ganglia. Damage to the putamen leads to a posture with flexion of the upper limbs and extension of the lower limbs,— the 'striatal position'. Extensive damage to the globus pallidus gives rise to a totally flexed posture, the 'pallidal position'. Transient dystonic postures and choreoathetotic movements may occur as a result of episodic failure of cortical control of the basal ganglia.

The pattern of most basal gangliar diseases changes from one of hyperkinesis to one of rigidity and postural fixation as the disorder progresses.

REFERENCES

[1] Albe-Fessard, D., Arfel, G., Guiot, G., Derome, P., Hertzog, E., Vourc'h, G., Brown, H., Aleonard, P., De La Herran, J. and Trigo, J. C. (1966). 'Electrophysiological studies of some deep cerebral structures in man.' *J. Neurol. Sci.* **3**, 37–51

[2] Barbeau, A. (1962). 'The pathogenesis of Parkinson's disease: A new hypothesis.' *Can. med. Ass. J.* **87**, 802–807

[3] Branch, C. L. and Martin, A. R. (1958). 'Inhibition of Betz cell activity by thalamic and cortical stimulation.' *J. Neurophysiol.* **21**, 380–390

[4] Brookhart, J. M. and Zanchetti, A. (1956). 'The relation between electro-cortical waves and the responsiveness of the cortico-spinal system.' *Electroenceph. clin. Neurophysiol.* **8**, 427–444

[5] Bucy, P. C. (1957). 'Is there a pyramidal tract?' *Brain* **80**, 376–392

[6] Carpenter, M. B., Strominger, N. L. and Weiss, A. H. (1965). 'Effects of lesions in the intralaminar thalamic nuclei upon subthalamic dyskinesia.' *Archs Neurol., Chicago* **13**, 113–125

[7] Cooper, I. S. (1961). *Parkinsonism. Its Medical and Surgical Therapy.* Springfield; Thomas

[8] Cooper, I. S. (1965). 'Clinical and physiologic implications of thalamic surgery for disorders of sensory communication. Part 2. Intention tremor, dystonia, Wilson's disease and torticollis.' *J. neurol. Sci.* **2**, 520–553

[9] Cotzias, G. C., Van Woert, M. H. and Schiffer, L. M. (1967). 'Aromatic amino acids and modification of Parkinsonism.' *New Engl. J. Med.* **276**, 374–379

[10] Denny-Brown, D. (1962). *The Basal Ganglia and their Relation to Disorders of Movement.* London; Oxford University Press

[11] Denny-Brown, D. (1966). *The Cerebral Control of Movement.* Liverpool University Press

[12] Duvoisin, R. C. and Yahr, M. D. (1965). 'Encephalitis and Parkinsonism.' *Archs Neurol., Chicago* **12**, 227–239

[13] Eadie, M. J. and Tyrer, J. H. (1965). 'Alimentary disorder in Parkinsonism.' *Australas. Ann. Med.* **14**, 13–22

[14] Ehringer, H. and Hornykiewicz, O. (1960). 'Verteilung von Noradrenalin und Dopamin (3-hydroxytyramin) im Gehirn des Menschen und ihr Verhalten bei Erkrankungen des extrapyramidalen Systems.' *Klin. Wschr.* **38**, 1236–1239

[15] Gastaut, H. and Fischer-Williams, M. (1959). 'The physiopathology of epileptic seizures.' In *American Physiological Society Handbook of Physiology.* Ed. by J. Field. Sect. 1, Vol. 1. Baltimore; Williams and Wilkins

[16] Gilman, S. and Van Der Meulen, J. P. (1966). 'Muscle spindle activity in dystonic and spastic monkeys.' *Archs Neurol., Chicago* 14, 553–563

[17] Greenfield, J. G. (1958). *Neuropathology.* London; Edward Arnold

[18] Guiot, G., Albe-Fessard, D., Arfel, G. and Derome, P. (1964). 'Dérivations d'Activités Unitaires en Cours d'Interventions Stéréotaxiques.' *Neuro-Chirurgie,* 10, 427–435

[19] Hodes, R., Peacock, S. M. and Heath, R. G. (1951). 'Influence of the forebrain on somato-motor activity.' *J. Comp. Neurol.* 94, 381–408

[20] Hoefer, P. F. A. and Putnam, T. J. (1940). 'Action potentials of muscles in athetosis and Sydenham's chorea.' *Archs Neurol. Psychiat., Chicago* 44, 517–531

[21] Jung. R. and Hassler, R. (1960). 'The extrapyramidal motor system.' In *American Physiological Society Handbook of Physiology.* Ed. by J. Field. Sect. 1, Vol. 2. Baltimore; Williams and Wilkins

[22] Kennard, M. A. (1944). 'Experimental analysis of functions of basal ganglia in monkeys and chimpanzees.' *J. Neurophysiol.* 7, 127–148

[23] Lance, J. W. (1963). 'Sporadic and familial varieties of tonic seizures'. *J. Neurol. Psychiat.* 26, 51–59

[24] Lance, J. W., Schwab, R. S. and Peterson, E. A. (1963). 'Action tremor and the cogwheel phenomenon in Parkinson's disease.' *Brain* 86, 95–110

[25] Landau, W. M., Struppler, A. and Mehls, O. (1966). 'A comparative electromyographic study of the reactions to passive movement in Parkinsonism and in normal subjects.' *Neurology, Minneap.* 16, 34–48

[26] Lessof, M. H. and Bywaters, E. G. L. (1956). 'The duration of chorea.' *Br. med. J.* 1, 1520–1523

[27] Lewin, R. J. and Porter, R. W. (1965). 'Inhibition of spontaneous bladder activity by stimulation of the globus pallidus.' *Neurology, Minneap.* 15, 1049–1052

[28] Li, C-L. (1956). 'The inhibitory effect of stimulation of a thalamic nucleus on neuronal activity in the motor cortex.' *J. Physiol., Lond.* 133, 40–53

[29] Martin, J. P. (1959). 'Remarks on the functions of the basal ganglia.' *Lancet* 1, 999–1005

[30] Martin, J. P. (1962). 'The negative symptoms of basal gangliar disease. A survey of 130 postencephalitic cases.' *Lancet* 2, 1–6

[31] McGeer, E. G., McGeer, P. L. and McLennan, H. (1961). 'The inhibitory action of 3-hydroxytryptamine, gamma aminobutyric acid (Gaba) and some other compounds towards the crayfish stretch receptor neuron.' *J. Neurochem.* 8, 36–49

[32] McMenemey, W. H. (1955). In *James Parkinson.* Ed. by M. Critchley. London; Macmillan

[33] Murnaghan, G. F. (1961). 'Neurogenic disorders of the bladder in Parkinsonism.' *Br. J. Urol.* 33, 403–409

[34] Oliver, L. (1958). 'The contributions of surgery to the treatment and understanding of Parkinsonism.' *Lancet* 1, 1121–1123

[35] Oliver, L. (1959). 'Parkinsonism due to midbrain compression.' *Lancet* 2, 817–819

[36] O'Reilly, S., Loncin, M. and Cooksey, B. 'Dopamine and basal ganglia disorders.' *Neurology, Minneap.* **15**, 980–984

[37] Poirier, L. J. and Sourkes, T. L. (1965). 'Influence of the substantia nigra on the catecholamine content of the striatum.' *Brain* **88**, 181–192

[38] Poirier, L. J., Sourkes, T. L., Bouvier, G., Boucher, R. and Carabin, S. (1966). 'Striatal amines, experimental tremor and the effect of harmaline in the monkey.' *Brain* **89**, 37–52

[39] Rand, R. W. and Markham, C. H. (1960). 'Hyperkinetic syndromes following thalamectomy and pallidectomy.' *Surg. Forum* **10**, 800–803

[40] Resnick, R. H., Gray, S. J., Koch, J. P. and Timberlake, W. H. (1962). 'Serotonin metabolism in paralysis agitans.' *Proc. Soc. exp. Biol. Med.* **110**, 77–79

[41] Richards, R. N. and Barnett, H. J. M. (1968). 'Paroxysmal dystonic choreoathetosis.' *Neurology, Minneap.* **18**, 461–469

[42] Selby, G. (1968). 'Cerebral atrophy in Parkinsonism.' *J. Neurol. Sci.* **6**, 517–559

[43] Stern, G. (1966). 'The effect of lesions in the substantia nigra.' *Brain* **89**, 449–478

[44] Stern, J. and Ward, A. A. (1962). 'Supraspinal and drug modulation of the alpha motor system.' *Archs Neurol., Chicago* **6**, 404–413

[45] Stevens, F. (1966). 'Paroxysmal choreo-athetosis.' *Archs Neurol., Chicago* **14**, 415–420

[46] Tardieu, G. and Tabary, J-C. (1965). 'Considerations sur l'Athetose de l'Enfant.' *Archs fr. Pediat.* **22**, 289–318

[47] Walter, R. D., Rand, R. W., Crandall, P. H. and Markham, C. H. (1963). 'Depth electrode studies of thalamus and basal ganglia.' *Archs Neurol., Chicago* **8**, 388–397

7—The Cerebellum and its Disorders

The cerebellum has a relatively uniform histological appearance and all parts appear to be fashioned to the same design with minor regional differences. However it may be considered in three parts on the grounds of developmental history, anatomical connexions and function. Each section forms part of a circuit regulating posture and movement, which may be regarded as a closed loop, embracing respectively the vestibular nuclei, the spinal cord and the cerebral cortex. It is as though the developing nervous system took advantage of an established co-ordination centre by ensuring that new projects were linked with the central computer as they developed.

DEVELOPMENTAL HISTORY

The cerebellum of invertebrates consists of a plate-like mass (*Figure 7.1a*), which develops in close association with the area receiving fibres from the labyrinth and lateral line[18]. In most groups of fish the cerebellum has two main parts, a caudal and basal vestibulo-lateral lobe which is connected with the labyrinth and lateral line, and a more rostral corpus cerebelli which receives fibres from the spinal cord, trigeminal nucleus and tectum. These two basic divisions persist in reptiles, birds and mammals (*Figure 7.1b*), although the lateral line disappears and the caudo-basal part of the cerebellum receives only vestibular fibres. In birds and lower mammals, the lateral parts of the cerebellum receive fibres from the pons, fore-shadowing the development in higher forms. In primates, the hemi-spheres of the cerebellum, which receive cortico-ponto-cerebellar fibres become progressively larger and more complex, in parallel with the growth of the cerebral cortex, as the phylogenetic scale is ascended (*Figure 7.1c*).

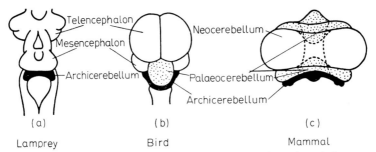

Figure 7.1. Developmental history of the cerebellum. The archicerebellum is associated with the lateral line in fishes and the vestibular system. The palaeocerebellum develops in connexion with spinal cord mechanisms. The neocerebellum appears as the cerebral cortex evolves and develops in parallel with it. (After Nieuwenhuys)[18]

ANATOMICAL CONNEXIONS

For convenience, the three divisions of the cerebellum are often referred to as the archi-, palaeo-, and neo-cerebellum in order of developmental seniority (*Figure 7.1*). The connexions of each division will be considered separately before discussing the integrative action of the cerebellum as a whole.

Archicerebellum

The flocculonodular lobe and adjacent uvula and nodulus is the vestibular part of the cerebellum[3]. This is phylogenetically the oldest part of the cerebellum and has reciprocal connexions with the vestibular nuclei via the inferior cerebellar peduncle (*Figure 7.2a*). This circuit is concerned with the maintenance of equilibrium.

Palaeocerebellum

The anterior lobe of the cerebellum and part of the posterior lobe, mainly near the midline, are dominated by impulses from the spinal cord[3]. Information is transmitted from the lower limbs by the dorsal and ventral spinocerebellar tracts. The equivalent pathways for the upper limbs, at least in the cat, are the cuneocerebellar and rostral spinocerebellar tracts[20]. The cuneocerebellar tract originates from the external cuneate nucleus, which is the equivalent in the cervical cord of Clarke's column in the thoracic and lumbar region, and corresponds to the dorsal spinocerebellar tract. Like the latter, it is uncrossed and enters the cerebellum through the inferior cerebellar peduncle. According to Oscarsson, the rostral spinocerebellar tract is the functional equivalent for the upper limb of the ventral spino-cerebellar tract in the cat, but, unlike this tract, it is uncrossed and enters the cerebellum through the inferior as well as the superior

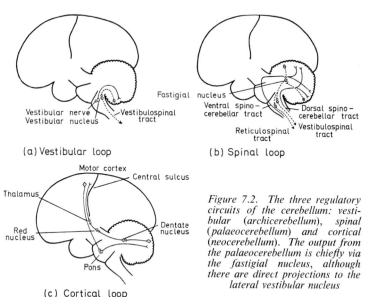

(a) Vestibular loop

(b) Spinal loop

(c) Cortical loop

Figure 7.2. The three regulatory circuits of the cerebellum: vestibular (archicerebellum), spinal (palaeocerebellum) and cortical (neocerebellum). The output from the palaeocerebellum is chiefly via the fastigial nucleus, although there are direct projections to the lateral vestibular nucleus

peduncle. The dorsal spinocerebellar tract originates from cells in Clarke's column and is almost entirely uncrossed. It carries information from ipsilateral group Ia and Ib muscle afferent fibres as well as from touch and pressure receptors and flexor reflex afferents of the same side. The ventral spinocerebellar tract arises from cells in the lateral part of the base and neck of the dorsal horn, which receive impulses from ipsilateral group Ib afferents and from flexor reflex afferents of both sides[20]. The ventral spinocerebellar tract is largely crossed in the spinal cord, but returns to the ipsilateral side of the cerebellum for its terminal distribution to the cerebellar cortex[20]. Synaptic transmission to spinocerebellar tracts is controlled by descending motor pathways, including the corticospinal tract. Spinocerebellar tracts end in both anterior and posterior parts of the cerebellum as mossy fibres.

There is also a slowly conducting spino-olivary tract, which is crossed, in the ventral columns of the spinal cord. The olivo-cerebellar pathway recrosses and terminates as climbing fibres in the cerebellar cortex. The significance of this relayed pathway will become apparent when the mechanism of cerebellar function is considered later.

The palaeocerebellum projects back to the spinal cord mainly via the lateral vestibular nucleus. Some fibres pass directly to the lateral vestibular nucleus, and others via the fastigial nucleus to the lateral vestibular nucleus of the same side. Other fastigiobulbar fibres pass to the opposite lateral vestibular nucleus by the hook bundle which arches around the superior cerebellar peduncle. There is a precise somatotopic relationship in the cerebellovestibular and vestibulospinal pathways, which permits the cerebellum to exert an influence on localized regions of the spinal cord, and hence on muscle tone controlled by alpha and gamma motor neurones in those parts of the cord[3]. There are also fastigioreticular connexions, which show no evidence of somatotopic organization. The palaeocerebellum thus influences reticulospinal and vestibulospinal pathways which regulate tone and posture through their connexions with the alpha and gamma efferent cells of the spinal cord.

Neocerebellum
The cerebellar hemispheres are linked reciprocally with the cerebral cortex, forming the third 'closed loop' of the cerebellum. Afferent fibres from the contralateral cerebral cortex are transmitted through pontine nuclei to the cerebellar hemispheres, and overlap to some extent near the midline with the cerebellar areas receiving spinal fibres. They end as mossy fibres.

Olivocerebellar fibres are also distributed to the neocerebellum, ending as climbing fibres. Efferents from the neocerebellum pass mainly to the dentate nucleus, lying in the white matter at the base of the cerebellum. The dentate nucleus projects to the red nucleus and the reticular formation surrounding it, and impulses are relayed from there to the ventrolateral nucleus of thalamus and on to the motor cortex. It appears as though descending activity in the great motor pathways is 'sampled' at the level of the pons by the neocerebellum, which can then modulate motor activity through the dentato-rubro-thalamo-cortical pathway.

THE INTEGRATING ACTION OF THE CEREBELLAR CORTEX

Although cerebellar connexions have been described as three separate circuits, there is considerable interaction between each. Indeed the histology of the cerebellum shows its potential for integration of activity in all areas of cerebellar cortex.

Afferent fibres from vestibular, spinal and cortical sources all terminate in the cerebellar cortex as mossy fibres, which synapse on granule cells. The axons of granule cells spread longitudinally as a dense beam of parallel fibres which activate Purkinje, stellate, basket and Golgi cells in the molecular layer[10]. The basket and stellate cells give rise to transversely running axons which inhibit rows of Purkinje cells on either side of the row which is excited by

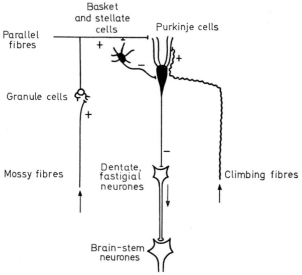

Figure 7.3. The integrating action of the cerebellar cortex. Mossy fibres excite granule cells which in turn excite a strip of Purkinje cells. The diagram also illustrates the way in which a zone of Purkinje cells is inhibited on each side of the excited strip, by means of basket and stellate cells. The climbing fibres from the inferior olive excite Purkinje cells and the degree to which they have been excited or inhibited by the mossy fibre input can be determined from their output. The Purkinje cells inhibit the lateral vestibular nucleus directly, as well as the basal nuclei of the cerebellum which normally exert both facilitatory and excitatory actions on the reticular formation and vestibular nuclei (after Eccles[9])

the parallel fibres. By this mechanism, any afferent input to the cerebellum via mossy fibres gives rise to a band of excited Purkinje cells flanked on each side by zones of inhibition (*Figure 7.3*). The degree of inhibition determines the responsiveness of Purkinje cells when they are stimulated by climbing fibres. It thus appears as though there is a dual system of projection from all areas to the cerebellar cortex consisting of mossy fibres, which bias or 'program' the

Purkinje cells and climbing fibres which sample the level of excitability of the Purkinje cells, thus reading out the stored information[9]. The mossy fibre pathway has a shorter conduction time by about 10 ms than the climbing fibres, which travel via the inferior olive.

It has been discovered that Purkinje cells are purely inhibitory in action[10]. They inhibit monosynaptically the basal nuclei of the cerebellum or Deiter's (lateral) nucleus of the vestibular complex in the brain-stem. The whole output of the cerebellar cortex is therefore negative in that it reduces the tonic discharges of these nuclei. The subcortical nuclei of the cerebellum have both facilitatory and inhibitory actions on the reticular formation and vestibular nuclei, which are thus modulated by the inhibitory control of the Purkinje cell output (*Figure 7.3*).

The organization of the cerebellum suggests that it functions as a servo-mechanism in the control of movement detecting and correcting errors of motor performance.

THE EFFECT OF THE CEREBELLUM ON SPINAL MOTOR SYSTEMS

Cooling or ablation of the anterior part of the cerebellum in the decerebrate cat reduces the activity of gamma motor neurones and increases the excitability of alpha motor neurones in the spinal cord[11]. Stimulation of the anterior lobe of cerebellum may inhibit or potentiate the monosynaptic reflex discharge of alpha motor neurones, depending upon the frequency of stimulation used[4]. In contrast to the variable effects on alpha cells, the great majority of all cerebellar stimulation sites enhance gamma efferent activity[16].

Complete removal of the cat cerebellum severely diminishes spindle activity in the acute phase, but some recovery occurs as the animal regains proprioceptive positive supporting reactions. Excitability of alpha cells is increased, at least in the acute phase[17]. After cerebellectomy, spindle activity is greater in flexors, which is reflected in the excessive flexion observed with movements such as forward stepping[22]. Cerebellectomy in monkeys gives rise to a flexed posture (dystonia in flexion) but this depends upon alpha cells, not gamma cells, since it persists after deafferentation of the limb[7]. In cats, extensor rigidity may develop, also mediated by alpha cell hyperexcitability (alpha rigidity). Denny-Brown and Gilman noted that a static tremor of the head and trunk appears 10–15 days after cerebellectomy in the monkey and is followed by a tremor of the limbs on movement[7].

149

The greater complexity of the human cerebellum and its close association with the cerebral cortex makes it impossible to explain entirely the effect of cerebellar lesions in man by extrapolating from the experimental animal. The phenomenon of alpha rigidity occurring after damage to the anterior lobe is rarely seen in man, in whom the end result of a cerebellar lesion is almost always hypotonia. How can this be so when the output of the cerebellar cortex is inhibitory?

The answer could be that the medullary reticular formation and some of the basal cerebellar nuclei exert a predominantly inhibitory influence on tonic mechanisms in man, so that the cerebellar cortex normally inhibits an inhibitor. Damage to the neocerebellum therefore permits unrestrained inhibition of gamma efferent activity by reticulospinal pathways. In contrast, the alpha motor neurone become hyperexcitable so that tendon reflexes remain brisk in spite of suppression of the gamma efferent system.

It has been suggested that gamma paralysis could be responsible for the incoordination and ataxia of the patient with a cerebellar syndrome. This is not so, however, because patients with gamma efferent paralysis from the intrathecal infusion of procaine do not have a cerebellar ataxia and are able to run their heel down the opposite shin with precision, even if a little uncertain in gait[15].

Experimental lesions in primates produce the most enduring deficit when they involve the neocerebellum, the lateral cerebellar nuclei (dentate and nucleus interpositus) or their efferent projection, the brachium conjunctivum. Growdon, Chambers and Liu[12] have recently investigated the effects of lesions of the lateral nuclei in monkeys trained to perform skilful acts. They found that cerebellar dysmetria and tremor are different aspects of a single deficit which is the result of the unregulated action of motor pathways, both pyramidal and extrapyramidal. They comment that the operated animals could often make a simple movement, such as taking food to the mouth, without ataxia or tremor. Once an error of rate, range or direction had been made, attempts at correction led to repeated errors until the goal was reached, when ataxia and tremor ceased.

The mechanism of dysmetria and intention tremor in man becomes apparent on deliberation. The cerebellum may be considered as a comparator or 'on-line computer' which regulates brain-stem mechanisms and the cerebral cortex in the smooth execution of voluntary movement. The feedback of proprioceptive and visual data about the position of the limbs in space is correlated with information concerning head position and the degree of motor activity so that corrective signals may adjust the movement of various parts of the body to conform with the pattern determined by the cerebral cortex. When this system breaks down, corrective signals have to traverse longer circuits and cease to be automatic. Each movement becomes a succession of jerky components. Over-correction is common so that a limb overshoots or oscillates about its mark.

THE SYMPTOMS AND SIGNS OF HUMAN CEREBELLAR DISEASE

It is possible to ascribe certain symptoms and signs of cerebellar disease to lesions of a particular part of the cerebellum[8] although the organ is often diffusely affected by disease, making analysis difficult.

Archicerebellar syndrome

The signs and symptoms of the archicerebellar syndrome are, (1) ataxia of gait; (2) vertigo and (3) nystagmus.

Involvement of the flocculonodular lobe by a discrete lesion, such as medulloblastoma in the child, or a secondary neoplasm in the adult, produces ataxia of gait as its earliest and chief manifestation, often accompanied by a sensation of vertigo and nystagmus. When the patient is tested in the lying position, heel–shin co-ordination may be unaffected. It is said that a lesion in the flocconodular lobe will protect an experimental animal against motion sickness, but there are simpler means of achieving this end in man.

Cerebellar nystagmus has the quick component directed to the side of the lesion. Positional nystagmus may be demonstrated by posturing the head backwards over the examination couch to the side of the lesion, in which case the nystagmus appears immediately and does not fatigue.

A rotated posture of the head is not uncommon with cerebellar tumours (*Figure 7.4*). The mechanism is not certain but probably depends upon damage to the vestibular system and its cerebellar projection.

Palaeocerebellar syndrome

The signs of a palaeocerebellar syndrome are, (1) ataxia of gait and (rarely) (2) alpha rigidity.

The cortex of the anterior lobe of the cerebellum is selectively affected in alcoholic cerebellar atrophy. This disorder is manifested by a broad-based gait with a tendency to lose balance and fall to either side. At first, co-ordination of the legs may appear normal when the patient is lying down, but difficulty in running the heel down the shin of the opposite leg is apparent sooner or later. Muscle

151

tone usually remains normal and the knee jerks are therefore not pendular.

The condition of alpha rigidity in which increased muscle tone depends upon hyperexcitability of the alpha cells, and therefore continues after gamma efferent block or dorsal root section, is rarely seen in man. Rushworth reported one instance of a patient with vertebral artery thrombosis in whom clonus persisted during procaine

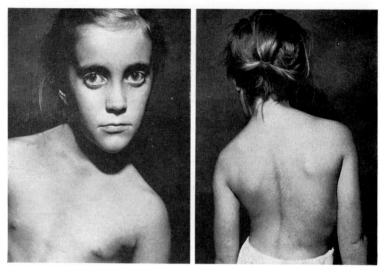

Figure 7.4. Abnormal posture of the head in a girl with a cystic astrocytoma of the cerebellum, leading to a compensatory thoracic scoliosis

block of the sciatic nerve until muscle power was grossly reduced[21]. Since procaine block reduces gamma activity before muscle power is lost, this was probably an example of alpha rigidity in man.

Neocerebellar syndrome

The following are signs of a neocerebellar syndrome. (1) hypotonia; (2) dyssynergia (delay in starting and stopping movements, rebound phenomenon, dysdiadochokinesia, decomposition of movement and speech, slurring dysarthria); (3) dysmetria; (4) static or postural tremor; (5) intention tremor; (6) ataxia of gait and falling to the side of the lesion; (7) nystagmus.

Hypotonia

Hypotonia is a constant feature of a neocerebellar syndrome in man. It may be detected in the posture of upper or lower limbs. A simple clinical test described by Sir Gordon Holmes[13], is to have the patient rest his elbows on a table and hold the forearms vertically with the wrist muscles relaxed. Normally, the hand makes an angle of about 30 degrees above the horizontal plane, whereas the hand of a hypotonic limb approaches the horizontal or sags below (*see Figure 4.2*). Diminished tonic reflexes can be sensed by the examiner manipulating the limbs through their full range of joint movement. When the thigh of the lying patient is rotated vigorously, the foot flails limply from side to side. Because the alpha system is normally active or hyperactive, phasic stretch reflexes remain brisk in cerebellar disease. Since the gamma system is underactive, the brisk reflexes are undamped by the tonic stretch reflexes, so that the knee jerks are seen to be pendular when tested with the legs dangling over the edge of the examination couch.

Dyssynergia

Dyssynergia is a term used to describe the disruption of the normal smooth control of movement provided by the graduated contraction of synergic muscles with relaxation of their antagonists. In cerebellar disease, voluntary movement takes longer to start and longer to stop. This may be demonstrated in a number of ways. The patient can be asked to lift both arms forwards rapidly and stop them when they are at 90 degrees to the trunk. The arm on the affected side will overshoot the mark and oscillate around the intended stopping point before coming to rest (*Figure 7.5*). When the patient is asked to pull against the examiner's hand, which is then removed suddenly, the patient's hand flies up and will strike his face if not prevented by the examiner's outstretched arm (*Figure 7.6*). This failure to brake a movement is known as a rebound phenomenon.

Difficulty in performing repetitive movements of the hands or feet rapidly are other manifestations of dyssynergia. Tapping or drumming the fingers on a resonating surface enables the dysrhythmia to be heard as well as seen. Alternating movements such as pronation–supination of the wrist are done slowly and clumsily. An increasing error in performance may become apparent, with the hand swinging more wildly with each sequence so that it flails in widening circles (dysdiadochokinesia). Movements lose their fluency in cerebellar disease and are broken up into their component parts (decomposition of movement). Turning disintegrates into a series of slow jerking movements ('turning by numbers') and speech is broken up into syllables ('scanning speech'). Because the art of speaking depends upon the fine control of movements of lips and tongue, speech is often slow and slurred in cerebellar disease.

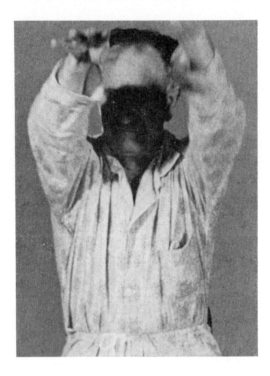

Figure 7.5. Delay in arresting movement in cerebellar diseases. The patient has been instructed to elevate the arms rapidly and stop them at 90 degrees to the trunk. The arm on the side of the cerebellar lesion overshoots the mark

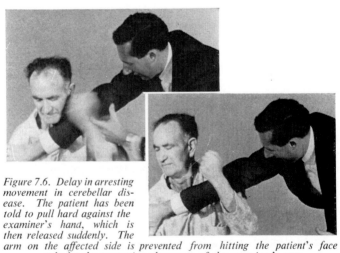

Figure 7.6. Delay in arresting movement in cerebellar disease. The patient has been told to pull hard against the examiner's hand, which is then released suddenly. The arm on the affected side is prevented from hitting the patient's face only by the protective placement of the examiner's arm

Dysmetria

Dysmetria describes the inability of the sensorimotor apparatus to measure distance in the course of a movement. Normally the smooth execution of a movement in which a limb is touched accurately to an external object depends upon constant feedback of information to the nervous system and correction of the movement in progress by cerebellar activity. In cerebellar disease, the limb may shoot past the object aimed at or deviate to one or other side, commonly to the side of the cerebellar lesion.

Tremor

A static tremor, or more correctly a postural tremor, may be evident in disorders affecting the dentate nucleus or its projection to the red nucleus and the reticular formation which surrounds it in the midbrain. The tremor which is most characteristic of cerebellar disease appears on attempting co-ordinated movement and is known as intention tremor. Intention tremor is an oscillating movement of the limb which becomes worse as the limb is advanced towards its objective, the oscillations taking place around the planned line of approach. The phenomenon is caused by delay in initiating and retarding correcting movements of the limb because of the absence of the neocerebellar servo-mechanism. The abolition of intention tremor by operative lesions placed in the ventrolateral nucleus of the thalamus is difficult to understand, but presumably depends upon blocking a faulty corrective mechanism.

Ataxia of gait, nystagmus

The gait is usually ataxic in neocerebellar disturbances and the patient tends to deviate to the side of the lesion in walking, and to fall to the side of the lesion.

It is uncertain whether nystagmus appears in lesions which are limited to lesions of the cerebellar hemispheres or whether this sign indicates impairment of the vermis and floccolonodular lobe. The eyes may show an oculomotor dysmetria in that there is consistent over-shoot of the eyes in moving from one object to the other[6].

DISORDERS OF THE CEREBELLUM

Developmental anomalies

Platybasia

Although platybasia is usually a congenital malformation in which the bone around the foramen magnum, with the atlas and axis, protrudes

155

into the posterior fossa, symptoms of cerebellar disturbance and hydrocephalus may not appear until adult life.

Arnold-Chiari malformation

A tongue of cerebellar tissue extends through the foramen magnum into the spinal canal, often associated with platybasia.

Agenesis and hypoplasia

Various unilateral and bilateral congenital defects of the cerebellum have been described.

Hypoxia

Hypoxia at the time of birth may give rise to a cerebellar deficit as one cause of the 'floppy baby syndrome'. Hypoxia in later life may also cause permanent cerebellar damage, often associated with myoclonus. Hypoglycaemia could theoretically produce the same result, although I have not seen any instance of its doing so.

Metabolic disorders

Myxoedema is of great importance as one of the potentially remediable causes of cerebellar ataxia[14].

Cerebellar signs may be present at some stage in Wilson's disease, and are seen in cerebral lipidosis, when they are commonly associated with myoclonic jerks.

Nutritional deficiency of nicotinic acid and riboflavin is said to produce a cerebellar syndrome.

An unusual familial disorder comprising relapsing cerebellar ataxia, a pellagra-like rash, and aminoaciduria, has been called Hartnup disease after the family in which it was first described[1]. It appears to be caused by an inability to produce nicotinic acid from tryptophan.

Hyperthermia may result in cerebellar atrophy.

Trauma

Head injury, particularly if repeated, may lead to a cerebellar syndrome as well as intellectual deficit and other cerebral changes (punch-drunkenness).

Injuries to the cerebellum by bullets and shell fragments provided much of the material studied by Sir Gordon Holmes as a basis for his classical description of cerebellar symptoms and signs[13].

Vascular disease

Insufficiency of the vertebrobasilar arterial system may produce transient or permanent cerebellar deficit.

Massive cerebellar infarction or haemorrhage into the cerebellum is uncommon, but may be fatal without urgent surgical decompression. The condition presents with sudden occipital headache, vertigo, vomiting and ataxia followed rapidly by impairment of consciousness.

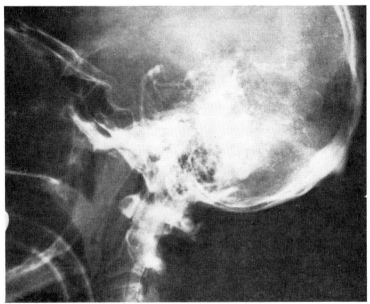

Figure 7.7. Angioma of the cerebellum, demonstrated by vertebral angiography, presenting with repeated episodes of subarachnoid haemorrhage and a unilateral cerebellar syndrome (patient illustrated in Figures 7.5 and 7.6)

Tumours
Angioma, haemangioblastoma, glioma and medulloblastoma are the commonest intracerebellar tumours. Fortunately most haemangiomata and gliomata in this site are cystic and the tumour contained within the cyst can often be completely removed surgically.

Vascular malformations of the cerebellum may be responsible for repeated subarachnoid haemorrhage (*Figure 7.7*).

Meningiomata, acoustic neurinomata and other posterior fossa tumours may compress the cerebellum.

Infections
It is well known that abscess formation may follow infections of the middle ear, and that diffuse involvement of the cerebellum may be

157

seen with encephalitis, for example, that of mumps or the exanthemata, particularly chickenpox. Myoclonus may be associated with a cerebellar syndrome following encephalitis.

It is not so well known that an acute cerebellitis may arise in children without any symptoms of generalized encephalitis or with no signs of infection, other than a non-specific upper respiratory tract infection. It is usually seen in a child between the ages of 2 and 4 years, and progresses over a few days. The picture is one of acute cerebellar disturbance, occasionally with headache and vomiting. The condition usually clears up in a few weeks, but may leave some residual symptoms for up to six months. The c.s.f. is usually normal, but slight increase in cells or protein may be found.

Intoxications

Alcohol produces an acute cerebellar syndrome with dysarthria, nystagmus, incoordination and ataxia. A similar picture may be seen with over-sedation by other drugs such as the barbiturates and Dilantin. The presence of a fine nystagmus can be used to check whether a patient on anticonvulsant medication is taking his tablets regularly. I remember one patient with a puzzling relapsing cerebellar syndrome who was eventually found to have a supply of barbiturates stored in a hollow celluloid doll which hung decoratively at the head of her bed

Lead, D.D.T. and other substances have been reported as causing cerebellar disturbance.

The continued intake of large amounts of alcohol may lead to a permanent cerebellar deficit[23].

Demyelinating diseases

Cerebellar signs are found in about 50 per cent of patients with multiple sclerosis.

Immunologically determined disorders

Cerebellar disturbance is commonly associated with rheumatic chorea, and is probably responsible for the hypotonia usually found in that condition.

Cerebellar degeneration has been reported in association with carcinoma, particularly of the lung and ovary[2]. The cause may be an auto-immune reaction, or the effect of some metabolic change produced by the tumour.

Familial cerebellar atrophy

Hereditary spinal ataxias

The spinocerebellar tracts are involved in Friedreich's ataxia, together with the posterior columns, pyramidal tracts and usually the peripheral nerves. A similar clinical picture may be found in ataxia-telangiectasia where cerebellar deficit is found in association with telangiectases on the conjunctivae, ear and elsewhere.

Cerebellar degeneration

Familial cases which have been reported can be grouped on pathological grounds under the headings of delayed cortical cerebellar atrophy and olivo-ponto-cerebellar atrophy, although clinically they are difficult to distinguish.

Familial myoclonic epilepsy

A progressive cerebellar syndrome is associated with myoclonus and grand mal epilepsy in one of the variations of familial myoclonic epilepsy, known as the Ramsay Hunt syndrome. It is transmitted by a recessive gene[19].

Sporadic cerebellar atrophy

From time to time one encounters patients with a progressive cerebellar syndrome which cannot be explained by any of the aetiological factors presented above. It is possible that some of these patients may have a chronic viral infection of the cerebellum. It has recently been shown that feline ataxia, which was previously considered to be a form of cerebellar hypoplasia, is caused by a virus. The suggestion has been made that human cerebellar disease may also be caused by a slow virus[5].

SUMMARY

The cerebellum has been described as a consortium of three systems, regulating vestibular, spinal and cortical mechanisms by means of reciprocal neuronal connexions. The histology of the cerebellar cortex indicates the way in which these three systems are integrated one with another. Recent work on the physiology of the cerebellum has demonstrated that each of the three divisions receives mossy fibres which 'program' the Purkinje cells and climbing fibres which 'read out' the stored information enabling the cerebellum to act as a servo-mechanism in the control of movement. The output of the Purkinje cells is inhibitory and cerebellar activity depends upon the projection pathways from the subcortical nuclei of the cerebellum, which have been modulated by the Purkinje cells.

Damage to the cerebellum is reflected in motor systems by increase in alpha cell activity and diminished gamma efferent activity, the combination giving rise to such clinical phenomena as the pendular knee jerk. The symptoms arising from damage to each section of the cerebellum are analysed separately and the nature of some clinical disorders affecting the cerebellum is outlined briefly.

REFERENCES

[1] Baron, D. N., Dent, C. E., Harris, H., Hart, E. W. and Jepson, J. B. (1956). 'Hereditary pellagra-like skin rash with temporary cerebellar ataxia, constant renal amino-aciduria and other bizarre biochemical features.' *Lancet* **2**, 421–428

[2] Brain, W. R. and Wilkinson, M. (1965). 'Subacute cerebellar degeneration associated with neoplasms.' *Brain* **88**, 465–478

[3] Brodal, A. (1967). 'Anatomical studies of cerebellar fibre connections with special reference to problems of functional localization.' In *The Cerebellum. Progress in Brain Research*, **25**, pp 135–173. Ed. by C. A. Fox and R. S. Snider. Amsterdam; Elsevier

[4] Calma, I. and Kidd, G. L. (1959). 'The action of the anterior lobe of the cerebellum on alpha motoneurones.' *J. Physiol., Lond.* **149**, 626–652

[5] Campbell, A. M. G. (1967). 'Feline and human ataxia.' *Lancet* **2**, 265–266

[6] Cogan, D. G. (1954). 'Ocular dysmetria; flutter-like oscillations of the eyes, and opsoclonus.' *Archs Ophthal., N.Y.* **51**, 318–335

[7] Denny-Brown, D. and Gilman, S. (1965). 'Depression of gamma innervation by cerebellectomy.' *Trans. Am. neurol. Ass.* **90**, 96–101

[8] Dow, R. S. and Moruzzi, G. (1958). *The Physiology and Pathology of the Cerebellum.* Minneapolis; Univ. of Minnesota Press

[9] Eccles, J. C. (1966). 'Functional organization of the cerebellum in relation to its role in motor control.' In *Muscular Afferents and Motor Control.* pp. 19–36. Ed. by R. Granit. Stockholm; Almqvist and Wiksell

[10] Eccles, J. C., Ito, M. and Szentágothai, J. (1967). *The Cerebellum as a Neuronal Machine.* New York; Springer

[11] Granit, R., Holmgren, B. and Merton, P. A. (1955). 'The two routes for excitation of muscle and their subservience to the cerebellum.' *J. Physiol., Lond.* **130**, 213–224

[12] Growdon, J. H., Chambers, W. W. and Liu, C. N. (1967). 'An experimental study of cerebellar dyskinesia in the rhesus monkey.' *Brain* **90**, 603–632

[13] Holmes, G. (1922). 'The Croonian lecture on the clinical symptoms of cerebellar disease and their interpretation.' *Br. med. J.* **1**, 1177, 1231; **2**, 59, 111

[14] Jellinek, E. H. and Kelly, R. E. (1960). 'Cerebellar syndrome in myxoedema.' *Lancet* **2**, 225–227

[15] Kjellberg, R. N., Todd, D. P., Schwab, R. S., England, A. C., Lance, J. W. and Sweet, W. H. (1961). 'Gait improvement in Parkinsonian patients by gamma motor neuron suppression.' *Trans. Am. neurol. Ass.* **86**, 126–130

[16] Manni, E., Henatsch, H. D., Henatsch, E-M. and Dow, R. S. (1964). 'Localization of facilitatory and inhibitory sites in and around the cerebellar nuclei affecting limb posture, alpha and gamma motoneurons.' *J. Neurophysiol.* **27**, 210–227

[17] McLeod, J. G. and Van Der Meulen, J. P. (1967). 'Effect of cerebellar ablation on the H reflex in the cat.' *Archs Neurol., Chicago* **16**, 421–432

[18] Nieuwenhuys, R. (1967). 'Comparative anatomy of the cerebellum.' In *The Cerebellum. Progress in Brain Research*, **25**, pp. 1–93. Ed. by C. A. Fox and R. S. Snider. Amsterdam; Elsevier

[19] Noad, K. B., Lance, J. W. and Walsh, R. J. (1960). 'Familial myoclonic epilepsy and its association with cerebellar disturbance.' *Brain* **83**, 618–630

[20] Oscarsson, O. (1962). 'Functional organization of the spino- and cuneo-cerebellar tracts.' *Physiol. Rev.* **45**, 495–522

[21] Rushworth, G. (1960). 'Spasticity and rigidity: An experimental study and review.' *J. Neurol. Neurosurg. Psychiat.* **23**, 99–118

[22] Van Der Meulen, J. P. and Gilman, S. (1965). 'Recovery of muscle spindle activity in cats after cerebellar ablation.' *J. Neurophysiol.* **28**, 943–957

[23] Victor, M., Adams, R. D. and Mancall, E. L. (1959). 'A restricted form of cerebellar cortical degeneration occurring in alcoholic patients.' *Archs Neurol., Chicago* **1**, 579–688

8—Vertigo

Vertigo is a common symptom and a most disturbing and unpleasant one. Vertigo may hide under cover of many sensations inadequately described by patients to their physician. Patients may complain of dizziness, giddiness, faintness, light-headedness, swimming in the head, or a feeling of 'everything going up and down'. It is not necessary to have the classical description of 'a sense of rotation'. The main complaints may be consequences of vertigo, for example nausea and vomiting, 'flickering of the eyes' (nystagmus), loss of balance, or falling attacks. The first step then is to make certain that the symptom from which the patient suffers is in fact vertigo.

Vertigo may be defined as a disorder of the awareness of the body's orientation in space. It may take the form of the ground moving up and down 'like a ship at sea', or a feeling of instability of the body in relation to surroundings. There may be a feeling of rotation, or of movement upwards or downwards. Anyone who, when retiring after an alcoholic evening, has experienced the terrifying illusion of a flying bed will realize how real, and how distressing, vertigo can be.

True vertigo is a symptom of disturbed function of the vestibular system or its central connexions. Because of the proximity of the vestibular end organs and nerves to those of the acoustic system, vertigo is often associated with tinnitus and deafness.

THE VESTIBULAR SYSTEM AND ITS CONNEXIONS

The vestibular labyrinth is divided into two parts, each of which provides a different type of information and mediates separate reflexes.

162

Perception of the position of the head in space; tonic reflexes

In a normal person, orientation of the head depends upon vision, labyrinthine mechanisms and body proprioceptors. A blindfolded cat can place its head in a suitable position in relation to gravity because of labyrinthine receptors. Conversely, an animal with damage to the labyrinths depends largely on the ability to see its surroundings. If an animal is both labyrinthectomized and blindfolded, orientation of the head and assumption of the upright position depends upon sensing the position of the body in relation to the environment by body contact and by joint receptors in the limbs. Head position is then adjusted to that of the body by receptors in the cervical spine and musculature and the tonic neck reflexes.

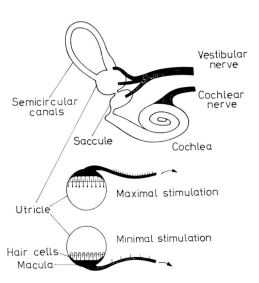

Figure 8.1. Schema of the internal ear, showing a stylized version of the otolith organ in the utricle. When the head is in such a position that otoliths hang from hair-cells, labyrinthine stimulation is maximal, as indicated by the vertical strokes (representing nerve impulses) superimposed on the branch of the vestibular nerve

The importance of the labyrinths and vestibular system in orientation was demonstrated by two of my patients whose vestibular nerves had been damaged, by streptomycin in one case and by vestibular neuronitis in the other. They separately described the experience of being submerged by a big wave while surfing and of opening their eyes while being tossed about under the water. Visual orientation was prevented by sand and foam in the turbulence of the wave and they had no idea of which way to swim to the surface. They were both eventually swept into shallow water in an exhausted condition.

The receptor responsible for signalling the position of the head is the otolith organ of the utricle in the internal ear. The utricle contains an end organ termed the macula, which is lined with hair cells covered with a gelatinous substance containing concretions of calcium carbonate. When the head is so placed that the weighted ends of the hair cells pull away from the macula, the vestibular neurones discharge at their highest frequency. Conversely, when the calcified tips of the hair cells are lying on the macula, vestibular

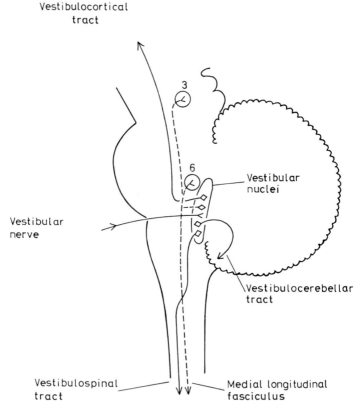

Vestibulocortical tract

Vestibular nuclei

Vestibular nerve

Vestibulocerebellar tract

Vestibulospinal tract

Medial longitudinal fasciculus

Figure 8.2. Some anatomical connexions of the vestibular nuclei. Fibres ascending to the nuclei responsible for eye movement in the medial longitudinal fasciculus take origin from all four of the large vestibular nuclei, and descending fibres from the medial nucleus only. The vestibulo-spinal tract arises from the lateral vestibular nucleus, in which cells are arranged somatotopically, thus permitting the effects of cerebello-vestibular connexions (not shown) to be distributed to localized areas of the spinal cord[2]

activity is least (*Figure 8.1*). These vestibular impulses pass centrally to the lateral vestibular nucleus in the medulla, where they influence muscle tone through the vestibulospinal tract, and are also transmitted to the cortex of the temporal lobe of the brain near the auditory area, so that the position of the head may reach awareness[7].

Perception of acceleration or rotation of the head

The appreciation of acceleratory or rotational movement is the function of the semicircular canals. The central projection of the vestibular system to the temporal lobe allows this information to be perceived. In addition, the vestibular system is linked closely with the vermis and flocculonodular lobe of the cerebellum for the maintenance of balance, and, through the medial longitudinal fasciculus, mediates eye movement and turning of the neck in response to movement of the head (*Figure 8.2*). The medial longitudinal fasciculus consists largely of fibres from the four main vestibular nuclei which run upwards to the nuclei of the third, fourth and sixth nerves, and fibres which run downwards from the medial vestibular nucleus to the motor neurones of the spinal accessory nerve and the anterior columns of the cervical cord[2]. This bundle of fibres is responsible for maintaining the visual axes parallel in lateral conjugate movement, as well as for tracking movements of the eyes necessary to maintain fixation of an object during head movement, and for turning of the neck to correlate with head and eye movements.

In health, the position of the eyes is adjusted from millisecond to millisecond so that clear vision is maintained even though the head is being jolted up and down or from side to side. The loss of this visual tracking mechanism is apparent when both vestibular nerves are damaged. A patient with bilateral vestibular damage will see objects clearly as long as the head is stationary. As soon as the patient walks or a vehicle in which he is travelling starts to move, objects appear to be jumping and blurred so that he can no longer read or recognize faces.

THE SYNDROME OF VESTIBULAR DAMAGE

The vestibular damage syndrome was described by Dandy after bilateral section of the vestibular nerves for Ménière's disease. It is seen nowadays after damage to the nerves from the toxic effects of streptomycin, or from vestibular neuronitis. It is characterized by the following.

165

Impaired balance and ataxia

The patient walks haltingly on a wide base in the same manner as a patient with cerebellar disease. This may gradually be overcome by practice and balancing exercises so that after a year or so the gait may be normal under good conditions of illumination. If lighting is poor so that the patient is deprived of visual orientation, he has to rely solely on proprioceptive mechanisms and balance again deteriorates.

The predicament of the submerged swimmer

The submerged swimmer's predicament is an extension of the above disorder in that visual orientation is impaired and tactile stimulation is uniformly distributed over the body while under water so that righting of the head becomes difficult or impossible.

Bus-rider's blurred vision

The inability to fix objects, read, or recognize faces when the head is moving up and down, ceases as soon as the patient's head is steady.

Interesting to relate, bilateral vestibular damage, once it is established, is not characterized by vertigo. If the patient was giddy at the onset of his illness, vertigo is lost once vestibular loss is complete.

NYSTAGMUS

Normally the eyes deviate laterally as the head is turned in order to maintain an object in the field of vision.

This reflex depends upon connexions between the vestibular nucleus and the centre for lateral conjugate deviation in the pons near the nucleus of the sixth cranial nerve. The reflex may be mediated by two neural pathways in parallel, the medial longitudinal fasciculus and a relay through the brain-stem reticular formation[7]. In a healthy subject, vestibular impulses from the semicircular canals tend to cause the eyes to turn to the ipsilateral side, but under resting conditions the vestibular input from each side is balanced so that the eyes remain stationary. If labyrinthine input becomes unbalanced by rotation of the head or by caloric stimulation, the eyes deviate slowly to one side then flick back rapidly to the point of fixation. The repetition of this sequence is known as nystagmus and the direction of nystagmus is conveniently designated by its fast component. Stimulation of the right medial or superior vestibular nucleus, or the left medial longitudinal fasciculus, produces nystagmus with a quick phase to the right[11]. In disease of one vestibular system (labyrinth, vestibular nerve or nucleus), nystagmus occurs when the eyes deviate to the side opposite the lesion because of the unopposed input from the healthy side. Because vestibular connexions with the cerebellum are predominantly crossed, nystagmus from a cerebellar lesion is usually directed to the side of the lesion. Vestibular nystagmus may be facilitated or inhibited by higher centres, a diencephalic centre situated between the lateral nucleus of the thalamus and the lateral geniculate body, and the cerebral cortex[11].

Nystagmus resulting from damage to the otolith organ of the utricle or its central connexions is produced by posturing the head backwards with the affected side underneath, for example, when the patient lies back in bed or looks suddenly upwards in the standing position.

The term optokinetic nystagmus is applied to the tracking movements of the eyes observed when gaze is maintained on a series of objects moving across the visual field, as when looking out from a moving vehicle. It may be tested by the subject watching figures on a rotating drum or on a strip of material drawn across in front of the eyes. Optokinetic nystagmus depends upon the integrity of the cerebral cortex in the vicinity of the supramarginal and angular gyri as well as the visual pathways. A lesion of the posterior temporal lobe or the supramarginal and angular gyri will cause a preponderance of optokinetic nystagmus to the side of the cerebral lesion (Carmichael, Dix and Hallpike[3]). The same authors showed that nystagmus induced by caloric stimulation showed a directional preponderance, that is, was sustained longer, to the side of the cerebral lesion when the eyes were open. When the eyes were closed, the electrical recording of nystagmus (electronystagmogram, ENG) showed that this directional preponderance was abolished or reversed[4].

Nystagmus commonly accompanies the symptom of vertigo.

The causes of vertigo

Vertigo is probably caused by imbalance between the input from the vestibular system of each side, or by abnormal patterns of vestibular impulses, or by conflict between visual, proprioceptive and vestibular information when one is inappropriate to the others. It is a symptom of breakdown of the complex 'orientating machine' described above, so that a sense of motion is experienced without adequate reason.

POSSIBLE SITES OF DISTURBANCE

External ear

Wax in the auditory canal is said to produce vertigo, but it is difficult to postulate a mechanism for this. I can remember only one patient whose vertigo ceased following the syringing of wax from the canal, and this may well have been coincidental.

Internal ear

Motion sickness

Motion sickness is the result of excessive labyrinthine stimulation.

Acute labyrinthitis

Usually, acute labyrinthitis is a sequel to Eustachian catarrh or otitis media, but may occur with viral infections. Vertigo is associated with tinnitus or deafness.

Haemorrhage into one labyrinth and internal auditory artery thrombosis

Haemorrhage into one labyrinth and thrombosis of the internal auditory artery both produce a sudden devastating vestibular failure with severe vertigo, tinnitus and deafness, and usually vomiting. Internal auditory artery thrombosis is often associated with vertebrobasilar insufficiency, so that acoustic symptoms may be bilateral and brain-stem symptoms or signs may be associated.

Labyrinthine fistula

Labyrinthine fistula is an unusual condition which may follow a mastoid operation[5].

Otosclerosis

Paroxysmal vertigo similar to that of Ménière's disease may be associated with the conduction deafness of otosclerosis[13].

Benign positional vertigo

A common syndrome, benign positional vertigo, is characterized by sudden giddiness on head movement, particularly on looking upwards or on lying down with the head turned to one side or the other. The disorder is caused by damage to the otolith organ and vertigo is produced when the head is postured backwards or when turned to the affected side. The condition is caused by otitis media, head injury or atherosclerotic changes in the internal auditory artery[9].

Ménière's disease

The commonest source of paroxysmal vertigo in adult life is Ménière's disease. Acoustic symptoms usually become added to bouts of vertigo, but remain unilateral in about 90 per cent of cases. Rarely, deafness may precede vertigo. The condition is associated with distension of the endolymphatic system and symptoms are produced by recurrent labyrinthine hydrops. The cause of this has not been established but vasomotor instability is thought to play a part.

Vestibular nerve

Infection

Vestibular neuronitis (epidemic vertigo) is thought to be a viral infection, and presents as acute vertigo without any acoustic symptoms. Vertigo gradually subsides but one or both vestibular nerves remain permanently damaged.

Benign paroxysmal vertigo of childhood is an episodic transient severe vertigo which recurs for some years without any acoustic or other symptoms developing. Caloric responses indicate a permanent deficit in vestibular function. The condition is probably a variant of vestibular neuronitis[1].

Toxins

Vestibular function may be impaired by salicylates, quinine or streptomycin. As little as 1 g of streptomycin will completely destroy vestibular function in an anuric patient and less than the normal therapeutic doses will damage the vestibular nerves in elderly patients, or in patients with renal insufficiency[6]. Alcohol and tobacco intoxication may cause a transient acute vertigo.

Compression

Tumours, particularly acoustic neurinoma, may cause a progressive unilateral nerve deafness with little or no vertigo, even though vestibular function is gradually abolished on one side. Neurinoma of the fifth cranial nerve, meningioma, cholesteatoma and an aneurysm in the cerebellopontine angle may have the same effect.

Brain-stem

Vertebro-basilar insufficiency

Transient ischaemia or infarction of the vestibular nucleus and its projection pathways to the cerebellum results from atheromatous changes in the vertebral arteries, the basilar artery or their branches;

or less commonly from compression of the vertebral artery by cervical spondylosis, or reduced filling pressure of the vessels in subclavian steal syndrome, or in 'hypotensive crises'. Vertigo is one of the most constant symptoms of vertebrobasilar insufficiency and is frequently associated with other brain-stem symptoms, or with impairment of vision from decreased flow in the posterior cerebral arteries. The tendency to vertigo is increased by anaemia or low cardiac output.

Migraine

'Basilar artery migraine' is a well recognized disorder in which symptoms of vertebrobasilar insufficiency precede or accompany a typical migraine headache, but last for 20–30 minutes, unlike the briefer episodes of ischaemia mentioned above. Vertigo is part of this syndrome and, in milder form, is experienced by about one third of all migrainous subjects in some of their attacks. The probable mechanism is transient vasoconstriction initiated by humoral changes.

Infections

Vertigo may be a symptom of brain-stem encephalitis or of meningo-vascular syphilis, which is now a rare condition.

Intrinsic lesions of the brain-stem

Multiple sclerosis, glioma and syringobulbia may cause transient or constant vertigo.

Cerebellum

The conditions mentioned above may affect the cerebellum or its connexions as well as the brain-stem.

Cerebellitis

An acute 'cerebellitis' may occur in virus infections, with vertigo as a prominent symptom. It may be seen as a complication of varicella. Cerebellar abscess may follow otitis media or rarely be secondary to pulmonary infection.

Tumours

Tumours of the cerebellum often present with vertigo, particularly of the positional variety. Central causes of positional vertigo may be distinguished by the onset of vertigo and nystagmus as soon as the head is placed backwards over the edge of the bunk with the head turned to the side of the lesion and the persistence of nystagmus as long as the posture is maintained.

Drugs

Drugs such as barbiturates, primidone, phenytoin and alcohol may cause vertigo with transient cerebellar dysfunction.

Cervical spine

It has been postulated that cervical spondylosis may cause vertigo by generating abnormal impulses from proprioceptors in the upper cervical spine, or by osteophytes compressing the vertebral arteries in the vertebral canal. The latter can be demonstrated by arch aortography or vertebral angiography, and may produce brain-stem symptoms when the neck is rotated sharply or extended. It is doubtful whether cervical spondylosis can cause vertigo in man through any other than a vascular mechanism, although nystagmus may be produced experimentally in rabbits by stimulation of the posterior cervical nerve roots[12]. Vertigo is not commonly associated with cervical changes, even when there is gross deformity of the upper cervical vertebrae, for example, in rheumatoid arthritis.

Eyes

The sensation of vertigo may be aroused by observation of any moving object which necessitates rapid tracking eye movements of nystagmoid type or by conflict of visual images as in diplopia.

Cerebrum

Electrical stimulation of the first temporal convolution gives only mild disturbances of equilibrium compared to the violent reactions obtained from stimulation of the labyrinth.

Temporal lobe epilepsy

Vertigo is an uncommon symptom of temporal lobe epilepsy but when it does occur, it is mild and associated with other hallucinations or illusions involving the special senses, emotions, memory or time-sense, or with automatisms which enable the diagnosis to be made.

Psychogenic vertigo

Psychogenic vertigo may depend on a sudden emotional reaction, for instance, on looking down from a tall building, or may be a more prolonged symptom of an anxiety reaction, often associated with overbreathing. In the latter form, it is worse when the patient is in a crowd or other situation which he or she may find distressing. There is commonly an underlying depressive state.

HISTORY-TAKING IN PATIENTS WITH VERTIGO

The following points are important to note

Pattern of vertigo (*Figure 8.3*)

Acute onset, gradually improving, for example, vestibular neuronitis, cerebellitis.

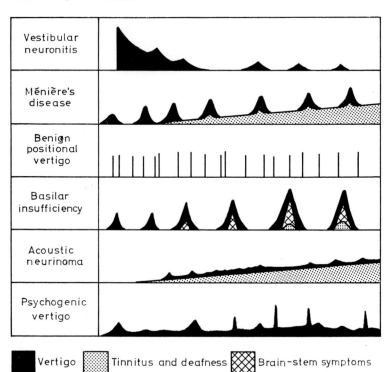

Vestibular
neuronitis

Ménière's
disease

Benign
positional
vertigo

Basilar
insufficiency

Acoustic
neurinoma

Psychogenic
vertigo

■ Vertigo   ░ Tinnitus and deafness   ▨ Brain-stem symptoms

Figure 8.3. Temporal patterns of various forms of vertigo. Vestibular neuronitis is of sudden onset and gradually improves. Ménière's disease is episodic and acoustic symptoms, usually unilateral, become added to vertigo. Benign positional vertigo is transient and recurrent, depending on head movement. Vertebrobasilar arterial insufficiency is episodic, and frequently associated with other brain-stem symptoms. The vertigo of acoustic neurinoma is superimposed on a progressive unilateral nerve deafness. Psychogenic vertigo is mild but persistent, with sudden exacerbations in stressful situations

Acute recurrent, for example, Ménière's disease, vertebrobasilar insufficiency.

Transient on head movement, as in benign positional vertigo.

Progressively increasing severity, for instance, eighth nerve tumour, central lesions.

Chronic, constant and ill-defined, as in psychogenic vertigo.

Associated symptoms

Tinnitus, deafness, for example, labyrinthitis, Ménière's disease, eighth nerve tumour, central lesions.

Transient bilateral visual disturbance or brain-stem symptoms, as in vertebrobasilar insufficiency, migraine.

Progressive or intermittent brain-stem symptoms, for example, posterior fossa tumour, multiple sclerosis.

Loss of consciousness, as in vertebrobasilar insufficiency, temporal lobe epilepsy.

Acute ataxia, incoordination, for instance, thrombosis, haemorrhage or infection involving cerebellum.

Progressive ataxia, incoordination, for example, cerebellar tumours.

Headache, for example, migraine, posterior fossa tumours.

Claustrophobia, anxiety and depression in psychogenic vertigo.

There may be no associated symptoms in vestibular neuronitis, early Ménière's disease or streptomycin toxicity.

EXAMINATION OF PATIENTS WITH VERTIGO

The tympanic membranes must be inspected and hearing tested in each ear by the whispered and spoken voice, the other ear being masked by a rapidly moving finger blocking the external auditory meatus. If hearing is impaired, tuning-fork tests determine whether it is of the perceptive (nerve) or conduction type. If a nerve deafness is severe in one ear, the tuning-fork applied to the mastoid bone behind the deaf ear may be heard in the other ear thus giving a false impression that bone conduction is better heard than air conduction in the affected ear.

The cranial nerves are carefully examined for nystagmus or signs of a brain-stem lesion. The corneal response and sensation to pinprick in the posterior wall of the auditory canal are checked on the side of a nerve deafness, since they may both be impaired by eighth nerve tumour, the latter because of compression of the sensory fibres in the nervus intermedius of the facial nerve (Hitselberger's sign).

Positional nystagmus is tested for by posturing the head backwards over the bunk from the sitting position, first to one side, then to the other. Peripheral causes (benign positional vertigo) give rise to vertigo and nystagmus after a brief latent period, which then subsides as the posture is maintained. Positional vertigo from central lesions comes on immediately the posture is assumed and does not fatigue.

Examination of the motor system may disclose hypotonia, pendular knee jerks, dyscoordination and ataxia if the cause of vertigo lies in the cerebellum.

A bruit over the neck may indicate stenosis of the vertebral arteries, and asymmetry of the radial pulses suggests the possibility of the subclavian steal syndrome.

SPECIAL INVESTIGATIONS

Caloric tests of vestibular function

The method of testing the caloric responses of the labyrinths described by Fitzgerald and Hallpike in 1942 is still in general use. The subject lies supine with his head flexed 30 degrees from the horizontal (a position which brings the lateral semicircular canal into a vertical plane) with his eyes fixed on a point above his head. Water at 30°C and 44°C (7° below and above body temperature) is used to irrigate the auditory canals in succession for a period of 40 seconds each. This sets up convection currents in the semicircular canal, which induces nystagmus. Nystagmus occurs with its fast component to the opposite side when cold water is used, and to the same side with warm water. The duration of nystagmus is timed from the start of irrigation of the canal to the end of observable nystagmus. The response is normally symmetrical and lasts from 90 to 150 seconds with both hot and cold water.

Two primary abnormalities may be distinguished by this test.

Canal paresis

A reduced sensitivity of one or both sides to both hot and cold water.

A unilateral canal paresis is almost invariably found in eighth nerve tumour, and is the most common abnormality in Ménière's disease. The change is unilateral or bilateral in vestibular neuronitis and bilateral in streptomycin poisoning (*Figure 8.4*).

Directional preponderance

The term directional preponderance is used to describe the unmasking of a latent imbalance in tonic vestibular mechanisms. To understand the result of the test, it must be appreciated that the use of cold water in the right ear, and warm water in the left ear, will

174

both cause nystagmus to the left. If these reactions are both greater than the corresponding reactions producing nystagmus to the right, the condition is termed a directional preponderance to the left.

Directional preponderance to the left is caused by a defect in the tonic vestibular system of the right side and vice versa. The tonic vestibular system probably comprises the utricle and its connexions with the caudal parts of the vestibular nuclei, inferior

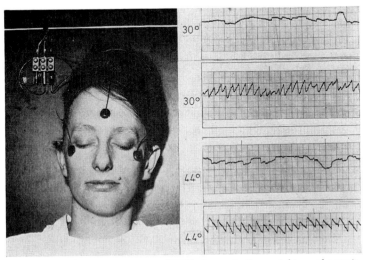

Figure 8.4. Electronystagmogram (ENG) demonstrating a right canal paresis. Electrodes are applied to the face as shown to record the electrical potentials produced by eye movement. Water at 30°C irrigating the external auditory canal evokes no response on the right (top tracing) and a normal response on the left (second tracing). Irrigation with warm water at 44°C again produces no response on the right (third tracing) and a normal response on the left (fourth tracing). (Photographs by courtesy of Dr. John Tonkin)

to the entrance of the eighth nerve. The primary defect with a lesion of the tonic system on one side is a slight deviation of the eyes which enhances nystagmus to the opposite side, thus resulting in directional preponderance to the opposite side[8].

Electronystagmography

Electronystagmography is a recording of spontaneous eye movements at rest or eye movements induced by caloric stimulation, based on the fact that there is a potential difference between anterior and posterior parts of the eye which sets up an easily recordable electrical potential on eye movement. This enables quantitative assessment of the intensity of nystagmus and separate measurements of its fast and slow component[14] (*Figure 8.4*).

Hearing tests

Audiometry[10, 15] provides a permanent quantitative record of hearing over a full range of frequencies and determines whether hearing loss is of the conduction or nerve type. In the case of nerve deafness, it is essential to distinguish between a peripheral or end-organ lesion such as that of Ménière's disease or a nerve lesion such as that caused by acoustic neurinoma. This can be done by the following tests.

Loudness balance test

The two ears are alternatively stimulated with the same frequency. The patient adjusts the intensity of sound heard in the good ear to that heard in the defective ear, and the procedure is repeated with differing intensities of sound presented to the defective ear. If the difference between the two ears is preserved at all levels of stimulus intensity, there is said to be no loudness recruitment, which is the case in disorders of the middle ear or eighth nerve (*Figure 8.5, a*). If the bad ear hears relatively better at higher intensities until it hears loud sounds as well as the good ear, loudness recruitment is said to be present, which indicates a cochlear lesion, usually Ménière's disease (*Figure 8.5, b*).

SISI (Short Increment Sensitivity Index) test

The SISI test determines whether a patient can hear small changes in sound intensity in the deaf ear better than in the normal ear. The ability to do this indicates that the lesion is cochlear. The normal ear usually hears from 0–20 per cent of changes of 1 db, whereas patients with Ménière's disease usually score 60–100 per cent at frequencies above 1000 Hz.

Békésy audiometry

The Békésy audiometer automatically increases the loudness of the tone at each frequency until the patient indicates by pressing a button that he hears the sound. The intensity of sound then decreases until the patient presses a button to indicate that he can no longer hear it. The frequency of the test tone is progressively increased through the full range and the patient's threshold is plotted at each frequency. The procedure is carried out twice, once with an interrupted tone and another with a continuous tone (*Figure 8.6*). The two curves are the same in normal ears, in middle ear disease, and

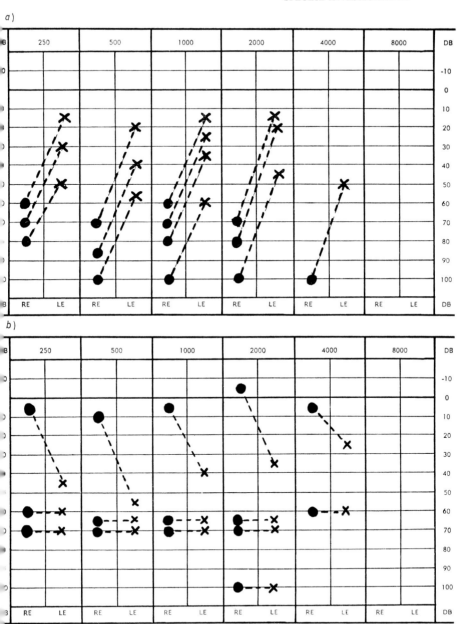

Figure 8.5. Loudness balance test. (a) Absence of loudness recruitment in a patient with acoustic neurinoma; (b) presence of loudness recruitment in a patient with Ménière's disease. (Chart photographs by courtesy of Mrs. D. V. Rockey)

5 per cent of cochlear disorders (Type I). The majority (95 per cent) of cochlear disorders show a slight falling off of ability to hear the continuous tone at high frequencies (Type II). Most eighth nerve disorders show a gross discrepancy between the two curves, with greater difficulty in hearing the continuous tone (Types III and IV).

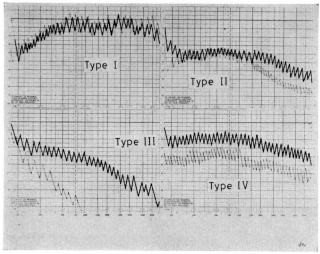

Figure 8.6. Békésy audiometry. The four types of response observed when testing with an interrupted tone (black line) and continuous tone (grey line). Description in text. (Photograph by courtesy of Mrs. D. V. Rockey)

Tone Decay

The test for tone decay is similar in principle to the Békésy test. A continuous tone is presented to the deaf ear until it can no longer be heard. The intensity is then increased by 5 db and the procedure repeated until 60 seconds have elapsed. If tone decay in this time exceeds 30 db, a neural lesion is suspected.

The commonest interpretation of these tests is as follows.

Deafness	Speech discrimination	Tone decay	Békésy	SISI	Recruitment
Cochlear	Fair	−	II (1)	+	+
Nerve fibre	Poor	+	III (IV)	−	−

DIAGNOSIS

A careful evaluation of the history, physical signs, caloric responses and hearing tests should make it clear whether the lesion is in the internal ear, eighth nerve, brain-stem or cerebellum. If an eighth nerve tumour or central lesion is suspected, radiography of the petrous temporal bones (Stenver's views) will demonstrate the internal auditory meatus. Tomography may be necessary to determine whether or not there is any expansion of the internal auditory meatus or erosion of the petrous temporal apex. Posterior fossa air studies or small-volume myelography can delineate the lesion precisely. The aim is to make the diagnosis of eighth nerve tumour while the deficit is limited to acoustic and vestibular symptoms, before there are signs of other neurological damage.

SUMMARY

Vertigo is an abnormal sensation of movement in relation to the environment and is commonly accompanied by nystagmus. It is a symptom of disorder of the vestibular system or its central connexions.

The vestibular system projects to the temporal lobe near the primary auditory cortex, and to the cerebellum. It is responsible for reflex movements of the head and eyes through the medial longitudinal fasciculus which links the vestibular system with the nuclei of the third, fourth and sixth cranial nerves and with the cervical spinal cord. The vestibulospinal tract alters muscle tone in relation to head posture and movement.

Tonic reflexes are mediated through the otolith organ of the utricle, which is also responsible for signalling the position of the head. Reflex eye movements and balance mechanisms are mediated through the semicircular canals, whose activity permits perception of acceleration or rotation of the head.

Damage to the vestibular system induces vertigo in the acute phase, and results in impairment of balance, disturbed righting reflexes in the absence of visual orientation, and the inability to maintain visual fixation when the head is moving. Each vestibular system tends to produce phasic deviation of the eyes to its own side, but under normal conditions, vestibular input is balanced. When one vestibular system is damaged, nystagmus therefore occurs to the healthy side, that is, the side opposite the lesion. Because vestibular connexions with the cerebellum are mainly crossed, the nystagmus of a cerebellar disturbance is directed to the side of the lesion.

The various causes of vertigo are considered briefly and an explanation given of tests of vestibular and acoustic function which are commonly used in the diagnosis of vertigo.

REFERENCES

1 Basser, L. S. (1964). 'Benign paroxysmal vertigo of childhood.' *Brain* **87**, 141–152
2 Brodal, A. (1963). 'Anatomical observations on the vestibular nuclei, with special reference to their relations to the spinal cord and the cerebellum.' *Acta oto-lar. Suppl.* **192**, 24–51
3 Carmichael, E. A., Dix, M. R. and Hallpike, C. S. (1954). 'Lesions of the cerebral hemispheres and their effects upon optokinetic and caloric nystagmus.' *Brain* **77**, 345–372
4 Carmichael, E. A., Dix, M. R., Hallpike, C. S. and Hood, J. D. (1961). 'Some further observations upon the effect of unilateral cerebral lesions on caloric and rotational nystagmus.' *Brain* **84**, 571–584
5 Cawthorne, T. (1957). 'Aural vertigo.' In *Modern Trends in Neurology-2*, pp. 193–201. Ed. by D. Williams. London; Butterworths
6 Cawthorne, T. and Ranger, D. (1957). 'Toxic effect of streptomycin upon balance and hearing.' *Br. med. J.* **1**, 1444–1446
7 Gernandt, B. E. (1959). 'Vestibular mechanisms.' In *American Physiological Society Handbook of Physiology*. Ed. by J. Field. Sect. 1, Vol. 1, pp. 549–564. Baltimore; Williams and Wilkins
8 Hallpike, C. S. (1966). 'The caloric test.' In *The Vestibular System and its Diseases* pp. 207–217. Ed. by R. J. Wolfson. Philadelphia; Univ. of Pennsylvania Press
9 Harrison, M. S. (1966). 'Benign positional vertigo.' In *The Vestibular System and its Diseases* pp. 404–427. Ed. by R. J. Wolfson. Philadelphia; Univ. of Pennsylvania Press
10 Jerger, J. (1962). 'Hearing tests in otologic diagnosis.' *Asha*, **4**, 139–145
11 Monnier, M. (1967). 'Central mechanisms of vestibular and optokinetic nystagmus.' In *Myotatic, Kinesthetic and Vestibular Mechanisms* pp. 205–218. Ciba Foundation Symposium. Ed. by A. V. S. de Reuck and J. Knight. London; Churchill
12 Philipszoon, A. J. (1967). In *Myotatic, Kinesthetic and Vestibular Mechanisms* pp. 195–198. Ciba Foundation Symposium. Ed. by A. V. S. de Reuck and J. Knight. London; Churchill
13 Richards, S. H. (1964). 'Ménière's syndrome in otosclerotics.' *Br. med. J.* **2**, 1227–1229
14 Stahle, J. (1966). 'Electronystagmography—its value as a diagnostic tool.' In *The Vestibular System and its Diseases* pp. 267–280. Ed. by R. J. Wolfson. Philadelphia; Univ. of Pennsylvania Press
15 Winchester, R. A. (1966). 'Audiologic patterns in vestibular disorders.' In *The Vestibular System and its Diseases* pp. 334–352. Ed. by R. J. Wolfson. Philadelphia; Univ. of Pennsylvania Press

9—Consciousness and Unconsciousness

What is consciousness? Although we all know exactly what is meant by the terms conscious and unconscious, definition is difficult. Consciousness is a state of awareness, in which the subject is capable of perception. A patient may be unable to interpret his perceptions, to correlate them with memory, to feel emotion, to think logically or to express himself by word or action, but if he is able to perceive by smelling, tasting, seeing, hearing or feeling, he is conscious. Consciousness may be considered as the state of activity in the brain which enables it to exert any of its functions as 'mind'.

The cerebral cortex is responsible for the content of consciousness but must be damaged severely and diffusely before producing loss of consciousness[16]. In contrast, a modest degree of damage to the midline structures of the thalamus and midbrain will produce impairment or loss of consciousness. The rostral part of the reticular formation may be regarded as the power supply for the complex computing system of the brain.

THE ASCENDING RETICULAR ACTIVATING SYSTEM

The cells of the reticular formation resemble motor neurones in appearance and are scattered throughout the brain-stem, enmeshed in fibres whose net-like pattern is responsible for the designation 'reticular'. The formation extends from the lower medulla, where it lies both laterally and posteriorly to the inferior olive, through the medial half of upper medulla and pontine tegmentum to the midbrain, surrounding the red nucleus between the third nerve nucleus and substantia nigra. The lateral reticular nucleus of the thalamus, the midline and intralaminar nuclei, and probably centrum

181

medianum, may be considered as the rostral end of the reticular formation as indicated in *Figure 9.1.*

The majority of reticular nerve cells divide into ascending and descending branches which link together the various levels of the reticular formation. The reticular formation receives afferent fibres from the ascending sensory tracts, vestibular nuclei, cerebellum,

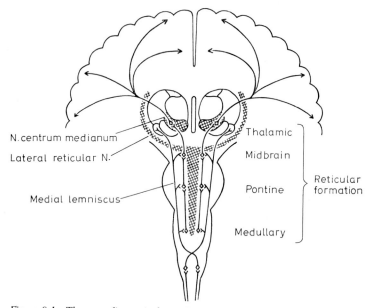

N.centrum medianum

Lateral reticular N.

Medial lemniscus

Thalamic

Midbrain

Pontine

Medullary

Reticular formation

Figure 9.1. The ascending reticular activating system. The reticular formation extends rostrally to include the lateral reticular nucleus of the thalamus, the midline and intralaminar nuclei, and part of centrum medianum, which project diffusely to the cerebral cortex as the unspecific afferent system, responsible for the maintenance of consciousness. The reticular formation of medulla, pons and midbrain receives collaterals from ascending specific sensory pathways

basal ganglia and cerebral cortex. Its main efferent projections are the reticulospinal pathways, which were described in Chapter 4, reciprocal connexions with the cerebellum and basal ganglia and the reticulocortical fibres. The reticular formation incorporates control centres for respiration, vasomotor tone, temperature and gastro-intestinal secretions.

Sensory fibres from the limbs, trunk and face, which are relayed in the posteroventromedial and posteroventrolateral nuclei of the thalamus pass to the appropriate areas of parietal cortex as the 'specific afferent system'. Repetitive stimulation of the specific sensory nuclei of the thalamus (VPM, VPL and ventrolateral nuclei) produce an augmenting response which is limited to the appropriate area of sensory cortex[17].

In contrast, reticulocortical fibres are distributed widely to most areas of the cerebral cortex as the 'unspecific afferent system'. Some reticulocortical neurones bypass the thalamus and others relay in the midline and intralaminar thalamic nuclei[6]. Although direct connexions with the cerebral cortex have not been demonstrated anatomically, repetitive stimulation of these thalamic nuclei, and of the nucleus ventralis anterior, rostral pole of centrum medianum and the lateral reticular nucleus evoke waves of activity which propagate diffusely over the cortex. These are known as 'recruiting responses' because they become progressively larger as stimulation is repeated[5]. Such recruiting responses are blocked when the brain-stem reticular formation is thrown into activity to produce an arousal reaction, suggesting that both phenomena are mediated by the same thalamocortical pathways[14].

It is possible that the midline and intralaminar nuclei and centrum medianum, which are involved in the recruiting response project to the nucleus ventralis anterior and the lateral reticular nucleus by short multi-synaptic connexions en route to the cortex[10].

In 1935, Bremer detected that the electroencephalogram (EEG) of an animal with a section made through the caudal end of the medulla showed a waking pattern. When a section was made through the upper midbrain, the EEG showed a sleeping pattern. Later Magoun and his co-workers found that stimulation of the central areas of the brain-stem reticular formation would transform the EEG from a sleeping to a waking pattern. These areas of the reticular formation and their rostral projections, which are responsible for arousal and for the maintenance of awareness, were therefore named the reticular activating system[13].

THE SOURCE OF CONSCIOUSNESS

Destruction of the midline structures of brain and brain-stem in experimental animals results in a state of akinesis and hypersomnia, resembling coma in man[7]. Stimulation of the intralaminar thalamic nuclei in unanaesthetized cats evokes a transient loss of consciousness resembling a petit mal 'absence' in man[9]. The implantation of irritant substances into midline areas of thalamus and reticular formation in immature animals has been used to induce absences experimentally.

183

Anencephalic infants display normal diurnal changes in consciousness if the rostral midbrain is intact, but not if it is involved in the congenital defect[15]. Injury to the upper brain-stem also demonstrates the importance of this region for the maintenance of consciousness in man. Compression of the midbrain by expanding lesions, such as tumour or subdural haematoma, leads to progressive impairment of consciousness[12]. The lesions of encephalitis lethargica, a disease which is characterized by somnolence, are distributed chiefly in the reticular formation of thalamus and midbrain[15]. Reduction of blood flow to the brain-stem reticular formation, caused by atheromatous narrowing of the vertebrobasilar arterial system or by vasoconstriction in 'basilar migraine', is commonly associated with alteration of consciousness, which is not the case when the source of transient ischaemic attacks lies in the internal carotid artery.

It is probable that most general anaesthetic agents act primarily on the reticular formation, since they block its activity at a time when conduction in the main sensory pathways is unimpaired[8]. Injection of amylobarbitone into the vertebrobasilar arterial system of man causes consciousness to be lost immediately, in contrast to the transient and inconstant impairment of consciousness when the common carotid artery is injected. Rosadini and Rossi concluded that consciousness was altered by the intracarotid injection of barbiturate when the opposite hemisphere was severely damaged, or when the injection filled the carotid circulation of both hemispheres, or when the drug entered the posterior cerebral artery which helps to supply the midbrain[18]. Stimulants such as the amphetamines are thought to act on the reticular formation to maintain awareness.

SLEEP

Why should we spend one-third of our life unconscious? The question is unanswerable at the moment. Although much is known about the mechanism of sleep, the nature of its restorative function is unknown.

The present hypothesis of sleep is that cortical neurones are influenced by inhibitory and excitatory centres in the thalamus, hypothalamus and brain-stem which hold the balance between sleep and wakefulness. The thalamic and midbrain components of the reticular activating system have been described. More caudal areas of the reticular formation, particularly in the rostral half of the pons, also play a part in the arousal response. Inhibitory centres have been described in the anterior hypothalamus and in the medulla around the tractus solitarius, which antagonize the reticular activating system[1]. Their destruction leads to a state of restlessness and insomnia.

The reciprocal relationship of neuronal systems for sleep and wakefulness is influenced by the barrage of afferent impulses from sensory pathways as well as by the cerebral cortex and by circulating humoral agents, such as adrenaline. The reticular formation receives collaterals from sensory tracts throughout its length and is responsible for a tonic activation of cortical neurones. A sudden incursion of sensory impulses produces temporary augmentation of reticular activity superimposed on the tonic background. Various afferent impulses which impinge upon it as the result of light, sound, bladder fullness and other sensations, summate in their effects to trigger the reticular activating system and awaken the sleeper.

Two phases of sleep may be distinguished on behavioural and electroencephalographic grounds. In normal sleep, runs of 15–18 c.p.s. activity are recorded in the EEG and are called sleep spindles because they wax and wane in amplitude. Later, slow waves at 2–4 c.p.s. appear bilaterally. Spindling is probably a function of unspecific sensory nuclei in the thalamus. Any sudden sound or arousal evokes sharp and slow waves recorded over the vertex, called a K complex. In deep sleep the subject lies still, there may be some contraction of neck muscles but no eye movements. This pattern of deep sleep is periodically interrupted by interludes of 'paradoxical sleep' lasting up to 15 minutes, often known as R.E.M. sleep because of the rapid eye movements observed or recorded at this time. Paradoxical sleep is characterized by fast low-voltage EEG activity similar to the normal pattern of arousal or alertness. It occupies about 15 per cent of normal sleeping time[11]. Nocturnal enuresis, sleep-walking and nightmares almost always occur at the stage of arousal from deep sleep[3].

LOSS OF CONSCIOUSNESS

Consciousness is impaired by failure of the reticular activating system or by diffuse disorder of the cerebral cortex. Causes of impaired consciousness are considered briefly here. Those requiring more detail are referred to a monograph by Plum and Posner[16].

Concussion

Sudden movement, or arrest of movement, of the brain within the skull produces a shearing strain across the midbrain which temporarily inactivates the reticular formation. The transient loss of consciousness which results is known as concussion. There have been other theories of concussion, such as waves of c.s.f. set up by the impact lapping through the ventricular system and breaking on the reticular shores, but the shearing strain hypothesis is most suited to the known facts.

185

Compression of the midbrain

Any enlarging intracranial lesions such as extradural and subdural haematoma, which displace the brain by external pressure, or intra-cerebral tumour and haemorrhage, which expand one hemisphere from within, can force a wedge of cerebral tissue downwards through the tentorial opening and compress the midbrain (*Figure 9.2*).

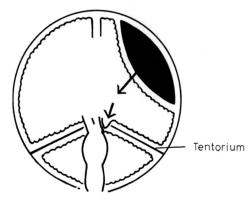

Tentorium

Figure 9.2. Tentorial herniation. Sketch showing the way in which an expand-ing intracranial lesion, such as a subdural haematoma, forces a tongue of cerebral tissue through the tentorial opening, compressing the midbrain and thus impairing consciousness

This process is known as tentorial coning or uncal herniation, because the uncus forms the tongue of tissue which is thrust through the gap between tentorium and midbrain. The third cranial nerve traverses this area as it runs from midbrain to cavernous sinus, and is stretched progressively during tentorial herniation, causing the pupil to dilate on the side of the lesion. Yawning and drowsiness give place to stupor and coma as the midbrain is compressed.

Compression of the brain-stem

Posterior fossa tumours may cause a reversed tentorial herniation, and block cerebrospinal fluid pathways as well as pressing directly on the brain-stem. Consciousness is lost, the pulse rate becomes slower, respiration becomes irregular and the patient may die from damage to medullary centres.

Drugs

Barbiturates and other hypnotic or anaesthetic agents exert their action by blocking synaptic activity in the reticular formation.

Cerebral infections

The drowsiness or stupor of encephalitis is caused by direct viral invasion of the reticular formation. The same areas may be rendered ischaemic in meningitis by interference with blood flow in perforating arteries at the point where they pass through the inflamed meninges.

Hypoxia

The reticular formation is supplied mainly by the basilar arterial system. Consciousness is lost in any condition which imperils the flow of blood in this system, or its oxygen content.

Hypoxia may be general as when oxygen-poor mixtures are inspired, or in airway obstruction, alveolo-capillary block or severe anaemia.

There may be inadequate filling pressure in the basilar artery because of low cardiac output. Loss of consciousness may result from pooling of blood in the periphery or splanchnic vessels as in simple fainting (vasovagal syncope), in states of surgical shock, or in patients who are given large doses of ganglion-blocking agents or other hypotensive drugs. Transient faintness is not uncommon when cardiac output is limited by stenosis of the mitral or aortic valves, or is suddenly reduced by cardiac infarction, intermittent heart block or a change in rhythm to atrial fibrillation or paroxysmal tachycardia.

Atheromatous stenosis of the vertebrobasilar arterial system may be the site of repeated platelet thrombi with episodes of embolization producing loss of consciousness together with other brain-stem signs. Apart from this, reduction of the arterial lumen may be sufficient in itself to impair blood flow, particularly when the blood pressure drops in one of the circumstances described above. Consciousness may be transiently impaired by vasospasm in 'basilar artery migraine'.

Hypoglycaemia

The brain metabolizes glucose as its chief, and perhaps sole source of energy. Hypoglycaemia therefore impairs cerebral function as rapidly and efficiently as hypoxia. If the fall in blood sugar is profound and prolonged, the brain is irreversibly damaged.

The most common cause of hypoglycaemic coma is administration of insulin to a diabetic patient in amounts which are excessive for his food intake. When food has been restricted by some intercurrent illness, often because of nausea or vomiting, the habitual dose of insulin may be sufficient to induce symptoms. In some diabetic patients hypoglycaemic symptoms may be induced while the level of blood sugar remains within normal limits, and on other occasions, the patient may remain conscious and alert at times when the blood glucose level is low. These anomalies may be explained by the brain having a glucose threshold which is sensitive to insulin, that is, after insulin, glucose can penetrate the brain at lower blood levels than before[4].

Hypoglycaemia may be produced by an insulinoma, or may occur as a reaction to the ingestion of glucose in post-gastrectomy or early diabetic states, or in response to L-leucine, galactose or fructose in susceptible infants. It may be symptomatic of liver disease or endocrine disorders, particularly Addison's disease and hypopituitarism[2].

The hypoglycaemic patient may complain of weakness, tremor and nausea before episodes of confusion, automatism or loss of consciousness.

Other metabolic disturbances
The use of glucose by the brain is impaired by lack of insulin and by ketosis in diabetic coma, by hypoxia and hypercapnia in respiratory failure, and by the accumulation of nitrogenous substances in renal and hepatic failure. All metabolic processes are reduced in myxoedema so that drowsiness or coma is accompanied by hypothermia. In hypopituitarism, the cause of coma may be hypoglycaemia, or secondary failure of the thyroid and adrenal glands. Thiamine deficiency, particularly liable to occur in alcoholics, affects the midbrain reticular formation in the syndrome of Wernicke's encephalopathy, which is characterized by ocular palsies, stupor and coma.

Epilepsy
Normal cerebral activity involves the asynchronous firing of nerve cells. In epilepsy, circuits of nerve cells fire repeatedly, with spread to adjacent cells until there is rhythmic activation of cortico-cortical or thalamo-cortical circuits. This may produce a transient loss of awareness such as the 'petit mal absence' or more prolonged unconsciousness associated with convulsions ('grand mal').

Hypothalamic lesions
The hypothalamus plays a part in the normal regulation of the sleep cycle by means of connexions with the midbrain reticular formation. Disturbance of hypothalamic function is usually associated with drowsiness or restless sleep clinically, although a state of undue wakefulness has been produced in animals by localized experimental lesions.

Narcolepsy
Narcolepsy is an increased tendency to sleep, which is presumably caused by a transient inhibition of the hypothalamic and brain-stem

alerting system, although the mechanism is unknown. The patient may sleep many times each day against his will, but awakens after some minutes feeling refreshed and able to carry on his normal routine. The appearance of the patient and EEG recordings are indistinguishable from natural sleep. The downstream reticular projections are often disturbed in narcoleptic patients in that the patient may be unable to move or speak for several minutes when in a relaxed or drowsy state (sleep paralysis) or may suffer attacks of physical weakness on laughing, sufficient to make him slump in his chair or fall to the ground (cataplexy).

CLINICAL EXAMINATION OF THE UNCONSCIOUS PATIENT

The appearance of the patient may be very helpful. The dry skin, flushed face and increased respiration of a patient in diabetic coma contrasts with the pale sweaty skin and quiet respiration of hypoglycaemic coma.

I remember an unconscious woman being carried into the casualty department. Her dry flushed skin, tachycardia and widely dilated pupils recalled a textbook description of belladonna (atropine) poisoning. A friend of the family confirmed this by describing how a relative living in the country had sent the patient some leaves with instructions to brew an infusion which would help her asthma. The patient made the brew, drank it, then lapsed into coma. One hour after the woman was admitted to hospital, her husband was brought to the casualty department in coma, with an identical appearance. The same distressed friend said that the husband had arrived home and was told that his wife had drunk a cup of tea and then lost consciousness. He said that this was a lot of nonsense and that nobody had ever become unconscious from drinking a cup of tea, and had then consumed a large glassful of the beverage. Happily, both recovered although the woman's asthma was little improved. Hyoscyamus alkaloids were demonstrated in the remaining tea.

Some insecticides contain long-acting anticholinesterase agents which may produce a clinical picture which is the reverse of that just described, with small pupils, pale sweating skin and muscular fasciculation. Barbiturate poisoning causes depressed respiration without any specific features.

Endocrine abnormalities may be evident on inspection, such as the dry skin and hair, and puffy face of myxoedema, the soft finely wrinkled skin and diminished body hair of hypopituitarism, or the pigmentation of Addison's disease. Spider naevi over the shoulders and arms, and palmar erythema point to the diagnosis of hepatic cirrhosis.

The depth of consciousness is gauged by the presence or absence of response to speech, touch, pressure and painful stimuli.

For those gifted with a good sense of smell, the breath may suggest the diagnosis of uraemia or diabetic ketosis. It should be unnecessary to mention that the smell of alcohol on the breath does not mean that alcohol is the cause of coma.

The scalp is inspected for signs of injury and the neck is gently flexed to test whether neck muscles are rigid from irritation of the meninges. A bruit may be audible over the orbits or mastoid processes in cases of intracerebral aneurysm or angioma, or in the neck, if one of the carotid arteries is obstructed. The fontanelles are palpated in infants. The fundi are inspected and the ears examined for signs of otitis media or haemorrhage from a fractured base of the skull.

The cranial nerves may be tested crudely in the unconscious patient. The size and symmetry of the pupils and their response to light is carefully noted. Eye movements may be tested by rolling the patient's head from side to side, which causes the eyes to deviate to the side uppermost if cranial nerves 3, 4 and 6 are intact (doll's eyes manoeuvre). The presence of a dilated pupil or other components of a third nerve paresis is of particular significance, since it may indicate impending tentorial herniation caused by a cerebral lesion on that side. Facial sensation may be examined by pinprick if the level of consciousness is sufficiently light to permit reflex facial grimacing. The symmetry of facial movement in response to painful stimuli, such as compressing the supraorbital nerve, will demonstrate a facial palsy of upper or lower motor neurone type. The pooling of secretions in the pharynx and the absence of a gag reflex may indicate involvement of the ninth and tenth cranial nerves.

Posture of the limbs and muscle tone on each side of the body should be contrasted. The limbs on a hemiplegic side fall heavily and tonelessly when dropped and will not move when painful stimuli are applied to the periphery. Reflex changes are noted carefully, with the emphasis on asymmetry. Sensation can be roughly estimated if any movement occurs with painful stimuli. The abdomen is palpated and percussed to assess whether the bladder is distended.

COMMON CAUSES OF COMA

When a patient is found in coma, the most common conditions to be considered are head injury, cerebral haemorrhage (including subdural and extradural haematoma), poisoning by alcohol or barbiturates, diabetic coma, hypoglycaemia and epilepsy. Other conditions mentioned above as causes of loss of consciousness must be considered since many of them, such as meningitis and Addisonian crisis, require immediate treatment, and others such as uraemia and myxoedema coma benefit from early recognition and treatment.

Coma is a medical emergency and often, as in the case of extradural or subdural haematoma, a surgical emergency. The deepening of coma, or the appearance of focal neurological signs, particularly a progressive third nerve palsy, is an indication for immediate action.

If there are no focal signs, and the cause of coma is not apparent after a rapid assessment, a useful measure is the injection of glucose intravenously following the withdrawal of a blood sample for glucose estimation. Intravenous glucose can do no harm, even in diabetic coma, whereas unrelieved hypoglycaemia can transform a patient into a decerebrate preparation in a matter of minutes.

SUMMARY

The midbrain reticular formation extends rostrally to embrace the midline and intralaminar thalamic nuclei as well as the lateral reticular nucleus and part of centrum medianum. Reticular areas of midbrain and thalamus project diffusely to the cortex as the 'unspecific afferent system', which is also known as the reticular activating system because its cortical connexions are responsible for maintaining a state of awareness. Certain areas in the anterior hypothalamus and in the medulla inhibit the reticular activating system and probably play an active part in the induction of sleep.

Consciousness is impaired when the rostral reticular formation is damaged by concussion, compression, drugs, infections, hypoxia, hypoglycaemia or other metabolic changes, or when its normal asynchronous activity is replaced by the synchronous discharge of epileptic paroxysms.

The neurological examination is modified in an unconscious patient so that the integrity of cranial nerves and motor and sensory systems may be assessed at least partially. Coma is a medical and surgical emergency, and its successful management depends upon understanding of the mechanisms involved.

REFERENCES

[1] Akert, K. (1965). 'The anatomical substrate of sleep.' In *Sleep Mechanisms. Progress in Brain Research* **18**, pp. 9–19. Ed. by K. Akert, C. Bally and J. P. Schadé. Amsterdam; Elsevier

[2] Beckett, A. G. and Samols, E. (1964). 'Carbohydrate metabolism.' In *Recent Advances in Medicine*, 14th Ed. pp. 105–147. Ed. by G. Beaumont and E. C. Dodds. London; Churchill

[3] Broughton, R. J. (1969). 'Sleep disorders: disorders of arousal?' *Science, N.Y.* **159**, 1070–1078

[4] Butterfield, W. J. N., Abrams, M. E., Sells, R. A., Sterky, G. and Whichelow, M. J. (1966). 'Insulin sensitivity of the human brain.' *Lancet* **1**, 557–560

[5] Dempsey, E. W. and Morison, R. S. (1942). 'The production of rhythmically recurrent cortical potentials after localized thalamic stimulation.' *Am. J. Physiol.* **135**, 293–300

[6] French, J. D. (1960). 'The reticular formation.' In *American Physiological Society Handbook of Physiology*. Ed. by J. Field. Sect. 1, Vol. 2, pp. 1281–1305. Baltimore; Williams and Wilkins

[7] French, J. D. and Magoun, H. W. (1952). 'Effects of chronic lesions in central cephalic brain stem of monkeys.' *Archs Neurol. Psychiat., Chicago* **68**, 591–604

[8] French, J. D. Verzeano, M. and Magoun, H. W. (1957). 'A neural basis of the anesthetic state.' *Archs Neurol. Psychiat., Chicago* **69**, 519–529

[9] Hunter, J. and Jasper, H. H. (1949). 'Effects of thalamic stimulation in unanaesthetized animals.' *Electroenceph. clin. Neurophysiol.* **1**, 305–324

[10] Jasper, H. H. (1960). 'Unspecific thalamocortical relations.' In *American Physiological Society Handbook of Physiology*. Ed. by J. Field. Sect. 1, Vol. 2, pp. 1307–1321. Baltimore; Williams and Wilkins

[11] Jouvet, M. (1965). 'Paradoxical sleep—a study of its nature and mechanisms.' In *Sleep Mechanisms. Progress in Brain Research.* **18**, 20–62. Ed. by K. Akert, C. Bally and J. P. Schadé. Amsterdam; Elsevier

[12] Magoun, H. W. (1950). 'Caudal and cephalic influences of the brain stem reticular formation.' *Physiol. Rev.* **30**, 459–474

[13] Magoun, H. W. (1952). 'An ascending reticular activating system in the brain stem.' *Archs Neurol. Psychiat., Chicago* **67**, 145–154

[14] Magoun, H. W. (1958). *The Waking Brain.* Illinois; Thomas

[15] Pilleri, G. (1966). 'The anatomy, physiology and pathology of the brainstem reticular formation.' In *The Brain-stem Reticular Formation and its significance for Autonomic and Affective Behaviour* pp. 9–78. Basle; Hoffman-La Roche

[16] Plum, F. and Posner, J. B. (1966). *The Diagnosis of Stupor and Coma.* Oxford; Blackwell

[17] Purpura, D. P. (1959). 'Nature of electrocortical potentials and synaptic organizations in cerebral and cerebellar cortex.' *Int. Rev. Neurobiol.* **1**, 47–163

[18] Rosadini, G. and Rossi, G. F. (1967). 'On the suggested cerebral dominance for consciousness.' *Brain* **90**, 101–112

10—The Mechanism of Epilepsy

Epilepsy is a recurring disturbance of cerebral function produced by paroxysmal neuronal discharge. The nature of the resulting seizure depends upon the area of grey matter where the neuronal discharge originates and the anatomical pathways along which it propagates. When the reticular formation of thalamus and midbrain is involved in abnormal activity, consciousness is lost.

The epileptic neurone
A study of the mechanism of epilepsy must start with consideration of single neurones and synaptic transmission. The cell membrane is normally maintained in a state of polarization, which depends upon the exclusion of sodium from the cell by an active metabolic process, the 'sodium pump'. The terminal boutons of other neurones are applied to the dendrites and cell body, and alter the polarization of the cell membrane by releasing a chemical transmitter substance which passes across the narrow synaptic cleft. Some transmitter substances cause hyperpolarization of the cell membrane, making the cell more stable and less likely to discharge, and are therefore called inhibitory transmitters. All inhibitory substances may be regarded as anticonvulsants, since they depress the tendency of neurones to discharge. Facilitatory or excitatory transmitters reduce the potential difference across the cell membrane. That is to say, they have a depolarizing action, and if a sufficient area of the cell membrane is depolarized, a chain reaction spreads along the entire cell membrane and the cell discharges. The only proven excitatory transmitter in the central nervous system is acetylcholine, which is released at synapses upon Renshaw cells in the spinal cord, and may be the transmitter substance for the ascending reticular activating system[5]. There is some evidence that L-glutamic and

L-aspartic acids may be transmitter substances in afferent and efferent central pathways respectively, and that noradrenaline, dopamine and 5-hydroxytryptamine may mediate transmission in a number of tracts radiating from brain-stem to cerebrum and spinal cord[5]. Glycine is probably the transmitter at those inhibitory synapses which are blocked by strychnine, chiefly in the spinal cord, whereas gamma aminobutyric acid (GABA) may serve as an inhibitory transmitter substance in the cerebral cortex and cerebellum[5].

If the net effect of synaptic influences upon a cell is facilitatory, it will be susceptible to discharge and transmit an impulse readily in response to excitation, possibly discharging repeatedly. Uncontrolled repetitive neuronal discharges, often synchronous with those of adjacent neurones, form the basis of the epileptic seizure.

The epileptic neurone is not simply an uninhibited neurone since its functional characteristics are altered. The potentials recorded from its soma and dendrites are of abnormally high amplitude and spread to the axons with greater frequency. Dendritic depolarization persists, so that epileptic spikes are readily generated by apical dendrites of the cerebral cortex[17].

There is still uncertainty about the manner in which a group of nerve cells become epileptic and form an epileptic focus, although many factors such as glial proliferation interfering with the normal metabolic processes of the cell, and isolation of areas of cerebral cortex from normal modulating mechanisms, have been considered[9]. Once a focus has formed it may remain localized, or its abnormal activity may spread to other areas of cortex, to the opposite hemisphere or to central structures. There is doubt as to whether central structures, the thalamic nuclei and reticular formation, are ever the primary cause of major seizures, or whether they are invariably provoked into epileptic activity by a cortical focus. The petit mal absence, on the other hand, with its accompanying bilateral 3 c.p.s. spike and wave pattern in the electroencephalogram, is thought to arise from central structures and has therefore been called 'centrencephalic epilepsy'.

The hereditary tendency to epilepsy

There are known genes for certain cerebral diseases of which epilepsy is a manifestation, such as familial myoclonic epilepsy, tuborous sclerosis and cerebral lipidosis.

The problem becomes more difficult when the importance of genetic factors is weighed against environmental factors in the production of grand mal seizures which are not the result of diffuse cerebral disorders. Metrakos and Metrakos compared the family history of children who were subject to convulsions with that of a control group[29]. They found that the prevalence of epilepsy in the relatives of the convulsant group was significantly higher, being three times that of the controls. If parents and siblings only were considered, the difference was even greater, 10 per cent of the convulsive group being affected, compared with 1·3 per cent of the control group. These data imply that children of a family with a low convulsive or epileptic threshold, are more likely to develop seizures as a manifestation of any systemic or cerebral disturbance. A patient with a hereditary low threshold may thus be more liable to suffer seizures as a result of birth trauma, cerebral infarction, brain tumour, or other cortical damage, than a patient with no family history of epilepsy. This view is consistent with the data of Lennox, who found a history of epilepsy in 3·6 per cent of the close relatives of those epileptic patients without any obvious brain damage, and 1·8 per cent of the relatives of epileptic patients with obvious brain damage, compared with the figure of 0·5 per cent for the general population[23].

In contrast to this rather vague concept of a convulsive threshold influenced by heredity, Metrakos and Metrakos were able to come to a definite conclusion about the inheritance of the 'centrencephalic trait'[30]. They used this term to include atypical spike and wave paroxysms in the EEG as well as the typical 3 c.p.s. spike and wave pattern, whether accompanied by major or minor seizures. The siblings of affected children were found to have centrencephalic EEG discharges in 37 per cent of cases. When the EEG was obtained between the ages of 4 and 16 years, 45 per cent of siblings were affected. When allowance is made for the tendency for this type of EEG abnormality to disappear in later years, the data are comparable with inheritance through an autosomal dominant gene. It was of interest that there was no significant difference between those patients with typical and atypical spike and wave patterns, and that only about one third of the children with EEG abnormalities had suffered overt seizures. Bray and Wiser have shown that a temporal lobe spike focus may also be an hereditary characteristic[3]. Of 40 families of epileptic patients studied, there was a close relative with a similar EEG focus in 30 per cent, and a close relative with bilaterally synchronous epileptic discharges in 48 per cent. The authors concluded that temporal lobe epilepsy could be inherited as a dominant pattern with age-dominant penetrance, reaching its maximum between the ages of 6 and 10 years.

In view of these recent genetic studies, it is surprising that the familial incidence of epilepsy is not more obvious in clinical practice.

From a practical point of view, one can advise epileptic patients in general that the chance of their having an epileptic child is about 1 in 36 if they marry a person without an epileptic history[22]. Occasionally one sees families with three or four epileptic children, a phenomenon which denies the odds quoted above. It is probable that in these families, the epileptic tendency is the result of a dominant gene such as the 'spike and wave trait' or 'temporal lobe trait' described above, or by a recessive gene such as that responsible for the rare condition of familial myoclonic epilepsy.

It has long been considered that there is an association between the inheritance of epilepsy and of migraine. A recent survey at this hospital of 500 migrainous patients and 100 patients who suffered from chronic tension headache, but were similar in ways other than the nature of their headache, disclosed that there was no significant difference in the personal incidence or family history of epilepsy between the two groups[21]. There was thus no evidence of genetic linkage between the two common hereditary paroxysmal disorders, migraine and epilepsy.

The consideration of epilepsy involves knowledge of the individual's predisposition to epilepsy, which probably depends upon the physicochemical control of neuronal discharge discussed earlier. The tendency to spontaneous epileptic discharge may be exaggerated by any form of cerebral damage or depression of inhibitory mechanisms.

FACTORS IN SEIZURE PRODUCTION

Failure of normal inhibition may be brought about by any circumstances which alter the distribution of sodium and potassium in the cell and the extracellular fluid, or selectively impair synaptic activity or the regulatory function of groups of neurones. These mechanisms have been summarized by Robb in his review of epilepsy[37].

Hypoxia and hypocapnia

Acute generalized hypoxia depresses first the cerebral hemispheres, releasing excessive activity in the brain-stem reticular formation which is then responsible for the convulsive seizure[11]. The sequelae of hypoxia include extensive damage to cerebral grey matter (including the deep layers of the cerebral cortex and cerebellum, the hippocampus and basal ganglia), which may permanently release control of the reticular formation, with the development of myoclonic jerks.

Local hypoxia may trigger convulsions in patients with cerebral vascular disease or during the vasoconstrictive phase of migraine.

Penfield and Jasper have shown that focal areas of cortical atrophy are surrounded by an area of relative ischaemia, which may thus be made susceptible to synchronous discharge[31]. Ischaemia is produced indirectly by overbreathing. Hyperventilation causes hypocapnia, which in turn causes cerebral vasoconstriction and cortical ischaemia. The technique of overbreathing is commonly used to demonstrate latent abnormalities in the electroencephalogram, since it accentuates any focal changes by increasing the degree of ischaemia surrounding a cortical lesion. The cerebral effects of hypoxia and hypocapnia are therefore additive, and the two techniques may be used together to determine the threshold of activation for any individual[36].

Hypoglycaemia

Since neuronal function depends upon metabolism of glucose, hypoglycaemia is tantamount to anoxia in its effects on the cerebral cortex. Hypoglycaemia is an important cause of convulsions, and may be provoked in infants by intolerance to fructose, galactose or L-leucine. Exogenous insulin, islet-cell tumours, hypopituitarism and adrenal insufficiency may be underlying causes in the adult.

Hyperthermia

The liability to convulsions from increased body temperature depends upon the genetic constitution of the individual and the rate at which temperature rises, as well as on the peak reached.

Electrolyte disturbances

Excessive cellular hydration or dehydration alters the shift of sodium across cell membranes. Adrenal insufficiency produces a diminution of potassium and increase in sodium within the neurone[44]. This partial failure of the 'sodium pump' mechanism leads to an increase in neuronal excitability. The changes produced in neuronal electrolyte balance by progestogenic hormones are less well understood, but are probably related to an increase in intracellular sodium in the premenstrual period.

Low serum calcium and magnesium levels increase neuronal excitability and may precipitate seizures.

Pyridoxine deficiency

Pyridoxine is essential for the activity of a decarboxylase responsible for the production of the inhibitor substance GABA from glutamate. Pyridoxine deficiency therefore lowers the brain concentration of

GABA and may provoke seizures. As the brain matures, the content of GABA progressively increases.

FACTORS IN SEIZURE PREVENTION

The normal nervous system contains many safeguards against excessive neuronal discharge. The liability of an individual to any form of epileptic seizure is referred to as the epileptic 'threshold'. A low threshold means that a nerve cell, or an aggregation of nerve cells, is prone to discharge more readily in response to some form of afferent stimulus. This in turn depends upon the degree of polarization of the cell membrane and the way in which it is altered by excitatory and inhibitory substances.

It is probable that anticonvulsant substances such as diphenyl-hydantoin act by enhancing the activity of the neuronal sodium pump, thereby increasing the membrane potential and stabilizing cell discharge. Acetazolamide (Diamox) produces a similar effect by inhibiting carbonic anhydrase, thus increasing intracellular carbonic acid, and reducing intracellular sodium.

Symonds described the variety of afferent stimuli which may initiate a seizure in a susceptible patient—visual stimulation by light or the complex act of reading, hearing simple sounds or musical tunes, touch of the skin or visceral sensations[41]. Sudden movement, or a startle reaction, or some kinds of mental activity may be sufficient to trigger the attack. In a normal subject, sensory or motor activity is contained within prescribed anatomical pathways and is limited to a period of asynchronous neuronal firing. This containment depends upon the cell membrane, synaptic transmitters, and the anatomical relation of inhibitory neurones. Transmission in afferent pathways is regulated at synapses by adjacent neurones and by descending motor pathways which depolarize the terminals of pre-synaptic neurones before they have the opportunity to pass on their message at the synapse. This pre-synaptic inhibition, as it is called, is a common mechanism at lower levels of the nervous system. At high levels—in the cerebral cortex, for example—post-synaptic inhibition is more common; that is, inhibitory neurones affect the cell membrane of the recipient cell, rendering it less excitable[8].

It is probable that whole groups of nerve cells, or nuclei, exert a constant inhibitory or restraining influence upon other nuclei, preventing their neurones from firing repeatedly in response to afferent stimuli. When such nuclei are destroyed, or temporarily put out of action, by anoxia or toxic agents, a local site of seizure discharge may develop in the area which was previously under

198

their jurisdiction. The localized hyperexcitability may be manifest as myoclonus limited in its expression to the movements of one limb, or may spread through devious anatomical pathways to produce a wider epileptic discharge.

THE MECHANISM OF SEIZURES

Tonic seizures

Tonic seizures, although rare, are interesting, because they may represent a single manifestation of epilepsy in isolation, although they cannot be classified definitely as epileptic in the present state of knowledge. A tonic (or dystonic) seizure is one in which the patient assumes an abnormal posture for some seconds or minutes. It is frequently unilateral, without loss of consciousness. The seizure may end without a clonic phase and without involuntary movements. The posture adopted is usually that associated with disorders of the upper motor neurone or basal ganglia—the 'striatal' or 'decorticate' posture, with flexion of the upper limbs and extension of the lower limbs. Such seizures were described in Chapter 6 as a transient dystonia, since the mechanism is probably one of temporary release of the basal ganglia from normal cortical control. The seizures are to be distinguished from decerebrate postures seen with diffuse cerebral disease, midbrain compression, or large cerebellar tumours.

Unilateral tonic seizures may be seen in conditions of generalized neuronal excitability, such as hypocalcaemia. They may also be superimposed upon pre-existing basal ganglia damage, or may appear in the course of multiple sclerosis, or as a symptom of a focal cortical lesion near the midline. Unilateral tonic seizures may also be a response to startle in otherwise normal subjects[18,25].

The preservation of awareness in some of these attacks demonstrates that the cerebral disturbance remains localized. The failure of a clonic phase to develop may result from the basal ganglia being implicated in the seizure discharge, as there is some evidence that inhibition of the tonic contraction in major epilepsy is initiated in the basal ganglia to bring about the clonic phase which is usually seen.

FOCAL SEIZURES AND MAJOR (GRAND MAL) SEIZURES

The division of major epilepsy into focal seizures arising in the cerebral cortex, and generalized seizures originating in the reticular formation of thalamus and midbrain (the 'centrencephalic system'), is currently being subjected to critical review.

The initiation of major seizures at a brain-stem or subcortical level is now thought to be rare. Williams has pointed out that large series of patients with cerebral tumours from the clinics of Cushing and Penfield show an incidence of fits with cortical tumours five times that found with tumours involving deep subcortical areas or the midbrain[42]. He speculates that major epileptic activity always

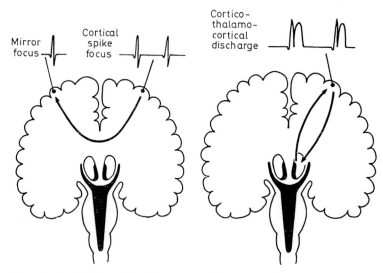

Figure 10.1. Focal cortical epilepsy. A potentially epileptic discharge may remain localized to one area of cortex, or propagate via the corpus callosum to the contralateral hemisphere, forming a mirror focus. Although such focal abnormalities are apparent in the EEG, the patient may remain free from seizures

Figure 10.2. Focal cortical epilepsy. A cortical discharge may spread locally through association fibres or extend to the reticular formation of thalamus and brain-stem (black areas in diagram). Such cortico-cortical or thalamo-cortical circuits are the probable basis of localized spike and wave patterns and overt focal seizures

starts in the cortex, and that involvement of deep structures by tumour may protect against seizures by destroying centrencephalic structures essential for generalized convulsions. Williams commented that disorders of the basal ganglia or operations upon the globus pallidus or the thalamus were not likely to provoke grand mal epilepsy. Attempts to induce epileptic foci in cat and monkey by injection of penicillin into medial and lateral thalamic nuclei have been unsuccessful, even when the dose used was five times the dose effective on the cerebral cortex[4].

The mechanism of focal seizures is at least partly understood. Local changes occurring in groups of cortical neurones as a result of isolation, ischaemia or changes in water and electrolyte content produce synchronous and repetitive neuronal discharges. Such discharges may remain localized, in which case they may not cause any symptoms, although they may be recorded as spike foci or focal seizure patterns on the electroencephalogram. Periodically, the epileptic disturbance may propagate to the corresponding point in the opposite hemisphere forming a 'mirror focus' (*Figure 10.1*).

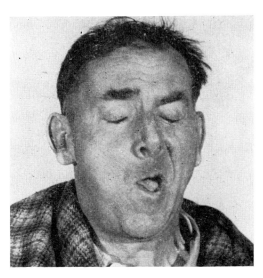

Figure 10.3. Focal cortical epilepsy. The left side of the face is seen to contract in the tonic phase of the seizure which was followed by a typical clonic phase. The patient's jaw was dislocated by the force of muscular contraction in each spasm, before the fits were controlled by intravenous diazepam

The discharge may also spread locally through short association fibres, involving progressively wider areas of cortex, or extend to the appropriate segment of the thalamus, setting up a thalamo-cortical circuit of impulses (*Figure 10.2*). In this case, the patient experiences a focal seizure, whose nature depends upon the area of cerebral cortex involved—hallucinations of the special senses, time sense, memory or emotion in the case of the temporal lobe, simple visual hallucinations of flashing points or zig-zags of light in the case of the occipital lobe, and paraesthesiae or involuntary movements of face or limbs when the sensorimotor cortex is implicated in the cortico-cortical or thalamo-cortical discharge (*Figure 10.3*). The focal seizure may be an event in itself, or may appear as an aura before a grand mal seizure. It may be restricted to one area of cortex, so that jerking of one limb or one side of the body may persist for hours (epilepsia partialis continuans) or may advance over the cortex, producing a 'march of symptoms' over the contralateral face and limbs (Jacksonian fit). Focal or partial epilepsy may extend to the medial thalamic nuclei bilaterally in susceptible patients, involving the reticular activating system in synchronous spike and wave discharges so that consciousness is lost (*Figure 10.4*).

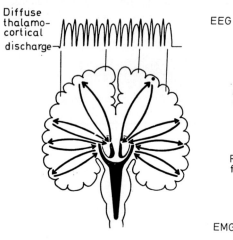

Diffuse thalamo-cortical discharge

EEG

Thalamus

Medical nuclei

Lat. retic. n

Reticular formation

Reticulospinal tracts

EMG

Tonic phase   Clonic phase

Figure 10.4. Diffuse thalamo-cortical discharge, associated with impairment of consciousness. This may be triggered by extension of epileptic activity from a cortical focus (secondary centrencephalic epilepsy) or may occur spontaneously in patients with the centrencephalic trait of petit mal epilepsy

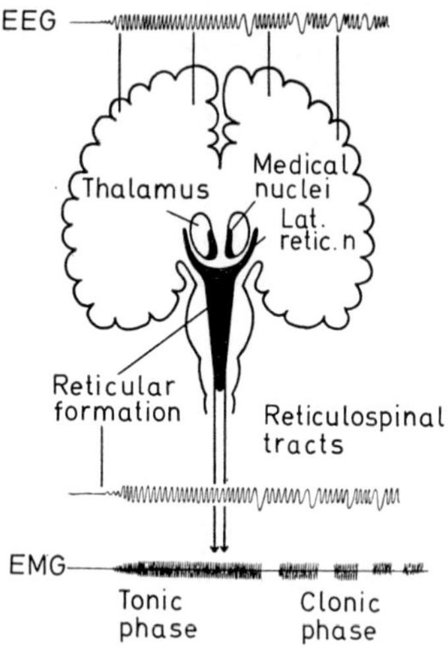

Figure 10.5. Grand mal seizure. The high-frequency EEG discharge of the tonic phase is later interrupted by slow waves which inhibit cerebral activity and permit brief periods of muscular relaxation, responsible for the clonic phase of the seizure

Not all generalized spike and wave discharges depend upon thalamo-cortical circuits. Stereotactically implanted electrodes in epileptic patients have shown that spike and wave discharges may be recorded from a variety of cortical sites without the participation of thalamic nuclei, although the form, rhythm and synchrony of the discharge is enhanced when the thalamus is involved in the paroxysm[38]. Experimental seizure discharges have been shown to pass readily to the contralateral hemisphere via the corpus callosum in cats whose thalamus, rostral hypothalamus and rostral midbrain had been destroyed[27]. It is apparent that a centrencephalic pacemaker is not essential for synchronous spike and wave discharges, which may propagate diffusely through the cerebral cortex along association fibres without involving midline structures.

Once a major seizure is established, the EEG pattern is one of bilateral high-frequency discharge (*Figure 10.5*). Both pyramidal and extrapyramidal pathways may conduct seizure activity to segmental levels of the spinal cord, which induces the initial tonic

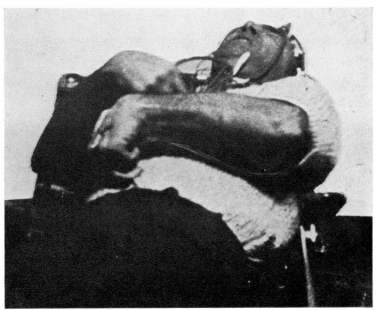

Figure 10.6. Tonic phase of grand mal seizure, showing flexed posture of upper limbs resembling tetanic spasm. (Photograph reproduced by courtesy of Dr. W. H. Wolfenden)

contraction of muscles, with the assumption of a rigid posture, commonly with arms flexed and legs extended (*Figure 10.6*).

The epileptic seizure is associated with an increase in cerebral oxygen consumption and CO_2 production, and there is some evidence of sodium loss and potassium gain by the brain[31]. The seizure is followed by severe cerebral and systemic acidosis. The termination of a grand mal seizure probably depends not only upon neuronal exhaustion by hypoxia and acidosis, but upon a positive process of inhibition. After some seconds of tonic contraction, during which high-frequency discharges may be recorded from cortex and subcortical structures, the patient relaxes intermittently, and this gives the appearance of the 'clonic' phase (*Figure 10.5*). The term 'clonic' is not strictly correct, since the phenomenon is simply a periodic interruption of the tonic phase. At the time of periods of relaxation, slow waves have been demonstrated in caudate nucleus and midline thalamic nuclei, with cessation of seizure patterns in the cortex. Jung postulated that these slow waves were 'braking waves' generated by the caudato-thalamo-cortical inhibitory system[11]. This concept is supported by animal experimentation, since Li found that single shocks to the ventrolateral nucleus of the thalamus arrested spontaneous activity in the motor cortex for periods up to 400 ms[24].

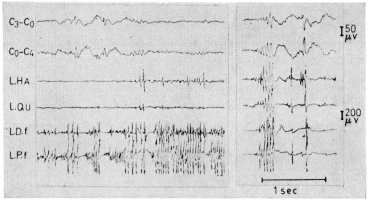

Figure 10.7. Correlation of EEG and EMG in myoclonus. The panel on the left shows cortical spike discharges preceding cortical slow waves and corresponding silent periods in the EMG. The panel on the right shows a series of cortical spikes augmented progressively until it gives place to a diphasic slow wave. A corresponding pattern is seen in muscular activity recorded from the leg, with increasing amplitude of myoclonic jerking followed by a silent period. EEG electrode placements are: left paracentral (C3), midline central (C0), and right paracentral (C4). EMG tracings are surface recordings from hamstrings (Ha), quadriceps (Qu), ankle dorsiflexors (D.f.) and plantar flexors (P.f.). (Reproduced from Lance and Adams[20] by courtesy of the Editor of 'Brain')

Intracellular recordings were made from cat cortex by Pollen while spike and wave complexes were generated by stimulation of the midline intralaminar system of the thalamus[35]. In most instances, the cortical spike was associated with excitatory post-synaptic potentials in cortical cells, and the surface-negative slow wave with inhibitory post-synaptic potentials, thus confirming the 'braking' nature of the slow wave.

In myoclonus, a similar slow wave is recorded from the cortex after a spike or spikes, and normal cortical activity is suspended for the duration of the slow wave. Muscle recordings in myoclonus show sudden shock-like contractions corresponding to the cortical spike or spikes in the electroencephalogram and an interruption of voluntary muscle activity or 'silent period' corresponding to the cortical slow wave[20] (*Figure 10.7*). During the silent period when muscle activity is suppressed, the patient may fall to the ground. The falling attacks of myoclonus are analogous to the periods of relaxation in the clonic phase of grand mal. The myoclonic jerk and falling attack therefore contain the components of grand mal. Gastaut and Fischer-Williams regarded the myoclonic jerk as an incipient grand mal attack which has been terminated abruptly by a process of active inhibition.

MINOR (PETIT MAL) SEIZURES

The petit mal 'absence' is a transient interruption of consciousness, lasting seconds only and recurring many times a day, sometimes every few seconds. It may be associated with flickering of the eyelids and brief automatic movements of the hands, and has been ascribed to a synchronous disturbance of the midbrain and thalamic reticular formation, although the factors necessary for its appearance are not understood. Flickering light is a trigger factor in some instances, and seizures may be self-induced by the patient rapidly passing his hand across his eyes in the sunlight. The same effect is obtained in a car driven along a tree-lined road with the sun slanting through the trees, and is procured artificially by stroboscopic stimulation during electroencephalographic recordings. Rhythmic 3 c.p.s. wave and spike thalamocortical activity has been elicited by stimulation of the intralaminar region of the thalamus by implanted electrodes in the unanaesthetized cat, which became immobile at the time in a manner resembling a petit mal absence[16]. Stronger stimulation precipitated a major seizure, with the recording of high-frequency discharges resembling those seen in the electroencephalogram during grand mal seizures in man. Guerrero-Fiqueroa and his co-workers reported the production of 'absences' in kittens by the implantation of alumina into the intralaminar nuclei of the thalamus and reticular formation[13]. The clinical attacks were associated with a 3 c.p.s. wave and spike pattern in the electroencephalographic record. Similar attacks could not be produced from other cortical or subcortical areas, and the technique was successful only if the implantation took place before the age of 30 days.

Although petit mal may unquestionably arise in central structures, there may be other patterns of spike and wave which radiate diffusely over the cerebral cortex without incorporating thalamus and mid-brain in the epileptic discharge, as has been discussed in the previous section[27,38].

MYOCLONUS

Myoclonus is an interesting epileptic manifestation, since it illustrates the principle that any neural system may become epileptic. A normal person given Metrazol will respond to sensory stimuli with myoclonic jerking.

Everyone is familiar with phenomena which resemble closely those of myoclonus, such as the startle response to a loud sound or unexpected tap on the shoulder, and the 'night start' which interrupts the steady drift into sleep. Indeed, night starts may recur so frequently in epileptic subjects that Symonds described the phenomenon as 'nocturnal myoclonus'[40]. Night starts may thus be an epileptic experience which, like the occasional déjà vu attack, is a reminder of the potential instability of the normal nervous system. The electromyogram during the startle response shows a waxing and waning of muscle activity similar to that seen in the symmetrical repetitive myoclonus of subacute sclerosing panencephalitis (inclusion body encephalitis) and some degenerative cerebral disorders, but quite different from the electromyogram of the more common form of myoclonic jerk, which shows a discharge of motor units as synchronous and clear-cut as a tendon jerk.

The relationship to myoclonus of the normal startle response (or of the related night starts on dropping off to sleep) has not been established, but these phenomena may well share a common mechanism. Bickford and his colleagues have demonstrated by computer-averaged electromyographic recordings that a subclinical muscle contraction occurs in normal subjects as a response to click stimulation and also to photic and somatosensory stimuli[2]. The photo-myoclonic response of epileptic patients has the same latencies and is probably an exaggeration of this normal muscular response (Broughton, personal communication). Dawson first drew attention to the fact that cortical responses to somatosensory afferent stimulation in myoclonic patients are similar in site and nature to those of normal subjects but are greatly increased in amplitude[7].

Myoclonus is a fragmentary manifestation of epilepsy, which may be of genetic origin, or which may be acquired as a result of diffuse brain damage, commonly as the result of hypoxia or encephalitis. The only instances of myoclonic jerking which I have observed to follow a discrete lesion of the brain are those of transient action myoclonus, which may be present for several days in the upper limbs contralateral to a stereotactic thalamotomy. It is of interest that Milhorat reported that destruction of the medial nuclei of the thalamus could produce myoclonus in the monkey[32].

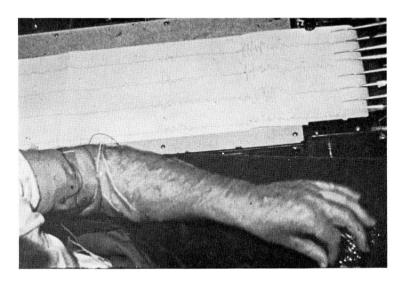

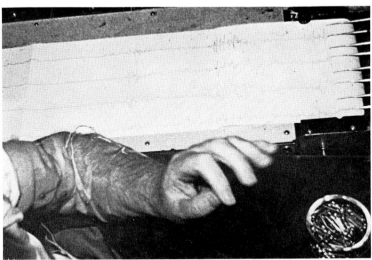

Figure 10.8. Action myoclonus. An attempt to retrieve a paper clip (a) produces a myoclonic jerk (b), the EMG of which can be seen in the polygraph recording

Myoclonus is a common accompaniment of major as well as minor epilepsy and may also be an isolated phenomenon without evidence of any other form of epilepsy, so that the term 'petit mal triad' to describe the association of myoclonic jerks and falls with petit mal absences implies a misleading specificity. Myoclonus is an expression of excitability of the nervous system, whose clinical manifestations depend upon the synchronous and repetitive firing of neuronal circuits in response to normal stimuli. It may be evoked by sound, light touch, tap or pinprick, as well as by attempted movement. It is most commonly seen in epileptic patients in the morning, when myoclonic jerking causes objects to fly out of the hands (*Figure 10.8*), and sudden jumping of the legs makes the upright posture hazardous. It is probable that a myoclonic jerk alone is not sufficient to cause a patient to fall, because balance can be recovered rapidly. The myoclonic state is usually associated with periods of inhibition of postural mechanisms (*Figure 10.9*), which often follow a myoclonic jerk and thus prevent a corrective involuntary or voluntary muscle contraction, so that the patient falls heavily to the ground (*Figure 10.10*)[20]. The myoclonic syndrome thus has two components, positive and negative. The myoclonic jerk is positive, in that the upper or lower limb is moved by a momentary active contraction of muscle; the falling attack is negative in that it is caused by transient inhibition of normal postural mechanisms, so that no muscular contraction is possible for up to one third of a second.

Myoclonic falling attacks are often attributed to clumsiness or carelessness, particularly in children, and their recognition as a neurological disorder may be long delayed. When they appear for the first time in a treated epileptic, they may be misinterpreted as the result of overdosage with anticonvulsants. In children they may be mistaken for habit spasms, the fidgeting of an anxiety state or rheumatic chorea.

Generalized myoclonic jerking may be seen during and immediately after an hypoxic episode; but, as the patient partially recovers, the myoclonic tendency becomes restricted to the limb or limbs which are involved in voluntary movement. This is particularly apparent with co-ordinated movements, and has been termed action or intention myoclonus[20,43]. The electroencephalographic changes in this condition are maximal on the side of the brain opposite to the limb undergoing myoclonic jerking, but nonetheless, multiple spike and wave patterns are propagated bilaterally. Lance and Adams considered that the clinical and electroencephalographic findings in this condition could best be explained by repetitive firing of

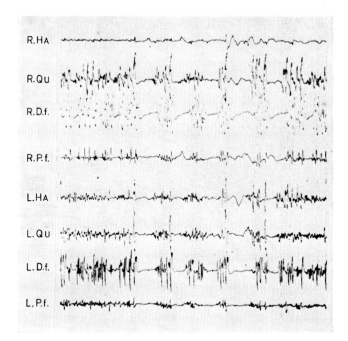

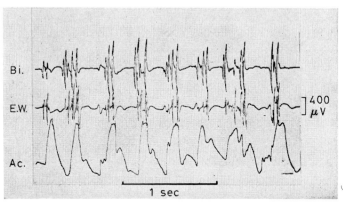

Figure 10.9. The mechanism of the myoclonic falling attack (inhibition of muscular contraction following myoclonic jerking). The upper panel demonstrates a silent period appearing simultaneously in the EMG of various muscle groups of both lower limbs after each myoclonic jerk. The lower panel illustrates the correlation between muscular activity in one arm and movement of that arm. The accelerometer output (Ac), direct-coupled to indicate displacement, shows how the limb falls downwards during the silent periods. EMG tracings are surface recordings from hamstrings (Ha), quadriceps (Qu), ankle dorsiflexors (D.f.) and plantar flexors (P.f.), biceps brachii (Bi) and extensors of the wrist (E.W.). (Reproduced from Lance and Adams[20] by courtesy of the Editor of 'Brain')

specific thalamocortical relays, whereas the bilateral rhythmic forms of myoclonus were more consistent with uncontrolled discharge of unspecific thalamocortical projections from the reticular formation. It is doubtful whether the myoclonic process is ever limited to any one grey matter nucleus or group of nuclei in man, because extensive lesions have been made in the ventrolateral nucleus of the

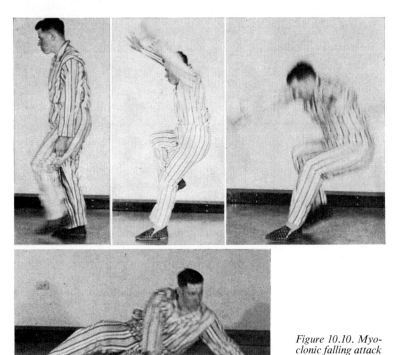

Figure 10.10. Myoclonic falling attack induced by startle

thalamus without preventing action myoclonus, although there have been instances of improvement following the procedure.

Myoclonus was divided into three categories by Gastaut and Rémond on the basis of electromyographic and electroencephalographic findings[12], and this neurophysiological approach is elaborated in the analysis by Halliday[15]. Type A is a brief shock-like contraction, sufficiently synchronous to look like a tendon jerk on electromyographic recordings. This corresponds to the clinical pattern of action or intention myoclonus described in the cerebellar form of familial myoclonic epilepsy[33, 43], and by Lance and Adams in post-hypoxic myoclonus[20]. It is the most common form of myoclonus, and occurs in idiopathic epilepsy, as well as in most myoclonus secondary to brain damage. The second and third types show the electromyographic recording of a normal muscle contraction ('interference') pattern and are usually rhythmic and bilateral. Type B is associated with infantile myoclonic spasms (jack-knife seizures), and type C with subacute sclerosing panencephalitis and some degenerative disorders. Halliday considers type A as 'pyramidal myoclonus' and types B and C as 'extrapyramidal myoclonus[14,15]. He adds another category, that of localized segmental myoclonus, found in virus diseases of the spinal cord or brain-stem. I recall seeing a cinematograph film of cats injected intraspinally with Newcastle disease virus by Luttrell and Bang[26]. The cats continued to have myoclonic jerks after decapitation, life being maintained by myoclonic inspiratory jerks. This was a convincing demonstration that myoclonus may be of spinal origin. The following classification of myoclonus is based on probable aetiology[19].

Genetic origin

(1) Idiopathic epilepsy, including hereditary essential myoclonus[6, 28].

(2) Familial myoclonic epilepsy, including the Lafora body type, system degeneration type and cerebral lipidosis[14].

(3) Tuberous sclerosis.

(4) Metabolic disorders such as phenylpyruvic oligophrenia, and Wilson's disease[43].

Acquired origin

(1) Hypoxia: (a) due to foetal or birth trauma; (b) other forms.

(2) Metabolic disturbances, including uraemia, hepatic encephalopathy.

(3) Intoxications, including organic compounds (such as methyl bromide) and drugs—for example, piperazine[39] and penicillin encephalopathy[10].

(4) Encephalitis, including subacute sclerosing panencephalitis, post-encephalitic syndromes and infections such as toxoplasmosis.

(5) Trauma, following head injury or stereotactic thalamotomy.

(6) Cerebral vascular disease in early childhood.

(7) Multiple sclerosis[1].

Syndromes of unknown aetiology: for example, infantile myoclonic spasms, cerebellar 'degeneration', Jakob–Creutzfeldt disease.

Localized segmental myoclonus: for example, spinal myoclonus, caused by virus infection.

In conclusion, myoclonus may be regarded as the motor expression of a general hyperexcitability of sensori-motor synaptic activity, so that response to any afferent stimulus is exaggerated, synchronous and often repetitive. If cerebral damage is minimal, the myoclonic tendency may be restricted to one limb, and brought out by activity of that limb (action myoclonus). If cerebral damage is more extensive, the response to any afferent stimulus may become myoclonic, and finally in severe generalized disorders, rhythmic, symmetrical jerking may become continuous in the absence of any external source of stimulation. There is no point in considering myoclonic jerks and falling attacks as part of a petit mal 'triad', since they are seen as often in association with grand mal seizures, or as isolated manifestation of epilepsy.

SUMMARY

Epilepsy is a recurring disturbance of cerebral function determined by the following factors.

(1) The genes: The petit mal absence, and some cases of temporal lobe epilepsy, may be inherited as an autosomal dominant characteristic. There is also evidence for the concept of a familial 'convulsive threshold', which renders patients more or less likely to seizures as a manifestation of any form of cortical damage.

(2) The cells: Depolarization of the cell membrane depends upon changes in electrolyte distribution between the cell and extracellular fluid. This may be altered by anoxia, hypocapnia, hypoglycaemia, hyperthermia, excessive hydration, dehydration, hypocalcaemia, adrenal hormones, progestogens, and anticonvulsants like the hydantoins.

(3) The synapses: Neuronal excitability is altered by excitatory and inhibitory transmitter substances released from nerve terminals on to the cell membrane. Anatomical safeguards are built into the nervous system in the form of pre-synaptic and post-synaptic inhibitory systems, to prevent repetitive firing of nerve cells. These may break down as a result of cerebral damage or toxic agents such as strychinine and Metrazol.

(4) The inhibitory neuronal pools: Certain collections of nerve cells normally exert a restraining action on other parts of the nervous system, and their destruction therefore causes synchronous and repetitive activity producing release phenomena, for example, myoclonus.

(5) Cortico-cortical circuits: Part of the cerebral cortex may form an epileptic focus as a result of ischaemia or by isolation from its

normal afferent connexions. Epileptic discharge may spread through surrounding areas of cortex by short association fibres or propagate to the opposite hemisphere via the corpus callosum.

(6) Thalamo-cortical circuits: Once synchronous discharge has been established in a part of the cortex, it may spread to involve thalamo-cortical connexions, initiating a focal or 'partial' epilepsy.

(7) Diffuse thalamo-cortical projections: Local thalamo-cortical discharge may become generalized if the cerebral threshold is low. When the whole of the reticular activating system is involved in the epileptic discharge, the patient loses consciousness.

(8) Descending motor pathways: Abolition of normal cortical control of the motor system, and the appearance of seizure activity in the reticular formation, produces tonic muscle contraction through both pyramidal and extrapyramidal tracts. The tonic seizure is usually interrupted after some seconds by an inhibitory process, which includes periods of relaxation known as the 'clonic phase' of a major fit.

Epilepsy may take the following forms.

(1) Focal cortical seizure: A localized cerebral discharge whose symptoms and signs depend upon the cortico-cortical or thalamo-cortical circuit involved, and which may be the 'aura' to a major seizure, or occur as an event in itself.

(2) Tonic seizure: The assumption of a transient dystonic posture, without a clonic phase, and usually without loss of consciousness, as a result of loss of normal cortical control of basal gangliar mechanisms.

(3) Major (grand mal) seizure: A tonic phase followed by intermittent relaxation ('clonic' phase), depending upon the reticular formation, but commonly triggered by a cortical disturbance.

(4) Minor (petit mal) seizure: Primary discharge of the reticular activating system resulting in transient loss of awareness.

(5) Myoclonus: Hyperactivity of any neuronal system (commonly manifested as jerking of the limbs) associated with episodes of inhibition of postural tonus (myoclonic falling attacks).

REFERENCES

[1] Aigner, B. R., and Mulder, D. W. (1960). 'Myoclonus. Clinical significance and an approach to classification.' *Archs Neurol., Chicago* **2**, 600-615
[2] Bickford, R. G., Jacobson, J. L. and Cody, D. T. R. (1964). 'Nature of average evoked potentials to sound and other stimuli in man.' *Ann. N.Y. Acad. Sci.* **112**, 204-223

[3] Bray, P. F. and Wiser, W. C. (1965). 'The relation of focal to diffuse epileptiform E.E.G. discharges in genetic epilepsy.' *Archs Neurol., Chicago* 13, 223–237

[4] Coceani, F., Libman, I. and Gloor, P. (1966). 'The effect of intra-carotid amobarbital injections upon experimentally induced epileptiform activity.' *Electroenceph. clin. Neurophysiol.* 20, 542–558

[5] Curtis, D. R. (1969). 'Central synaptic transmitters.' In *Basic Mechanisms of the Epilepsies*. Ed. by H. H. Jasper. Boston; Little, Brown

[6] Daube, J. R. and Peters, H. A. (1966). 'Hereditary essential myoclonus.' *Archs Neurol. Chicago* 15, 587–594

[7] Dawson, G. D. (1947). 'Investigations on a patient subject to myoclonic seizures after sensory stimulation.' *J. Neurol. Neurosurg. Psychiat.* 10, 141–162

[8] Eccles, J. C. (1964). *The Physiology of Synapses* pp. 233–234. Berlin; Springer

[9] Echlin, F. A. and Battista, A. (1963). 'Epileptiform seizures from chronic isolated cortex.' *Archs Neurol., Chicago* 9, 154–170

[10] Editorial. (1967). 'Penicillin encephalopathy.' *Br. med. J.* 2, 384

[11] Gastaut, H. and Fischer-Williams, M. (1959). 'The physiopathology of epileptic seizures.' In *American Physiological Society Handbook of Physiology*. Sect. 1, Vol. 1, pp. 329–363. Baltimore; Williams and Wilkins

[12] Gastaut, H. and Rémond, A. (1952). 'Étude électroéncephalographique des myoclonies.' *Revue Neurol.* 86, 596–609

[13] Guerrero-Fiqueroa, R., Barros, A., De Balbian Verster, F. and Heath, R. G. (1963). 'Experimental "petit mal" in kittens.' *Archs Neurol. Chicago* 9, 297–306

[14] Halliday, A. M. (1967). 'The clinical incidence of myoclonus.' In *Modern Trends in Neurology*-4 pp. 69–105. Ed. by D. Williams. London; Butterworths

[15] Halliday, A. M. (1967). 'The electrophysiological study of myoclonus in man.' *Brain* 90, 241–284

[16] Hunter, J. and Jasper, H. H. (1949). 'Effects of thalamic stimulation in unanaesthetized animals: the arrest reaction and petit mal-like seizures, activation patterns and generalized convulsions.' *Electroenceph. clin. Neurophysiol.* 1, 305–324

[17] Kreindler, A. (1965). *Experimental Epilepsy. Progress in Brain Research*. Amsterdam; Elsevier

[18] Lance, J. W. (1963). 'Sporadic and familial varieties of tonic seizures.' *J. Neurol. Neurosurg. Psychiat.* 26, 51–59

[19] Lance, J. W. (1968). 'Myoclonic jerks and falls: aetiology, classification and treatment.' *Med. J. Aust.* 1, 113–120

[20] Lance, J. W. and Adams, R. D. (1963). 'The syndrome of intention or action myoclonus as a sequel to hypoxic encephalopathy.' *Brain* 86, 111–136

[21] Lance, J. W. and Anthony, M. (1966). 'Some clinical aspects of migraine.' *Archs Neurol., Chicago* 15, 356–361

[22] Lennox, W. G. (1941). *Science and Seizures*. New York; Harper

[23] Lennox, W. G. (1951). 'The heredity of epilepsy as told by relatives and twins.' *J. Am. med. Ass.* 146, 529–536

[24] Li, C. L. (1956). 'The inhibitory effect of stimulation of a thalamic nucleus on neuronal activity in the motor cortex.' *J. Physiol., Lond.* **133**, 40–53

[25] Lishman, W. A., Symonds, C. P., Whitty, C. W. M. and Willison, R. G. (1962). 'Seizures induced by movement.' *Brain* **85**, 93–108

[26] Luttrell, C. N. and Bang, F. B. (1959). 'Newcastle disease encephalomyelitis in cats II. Physiological studies on rhythmic myoclonus.' *Archs Neurol. Psychiat., Chicago* **81**, 285–291

[27] Marcus, E. M. and Watson, C. W. (1966). 'Bilateral synchronous spike wave electrographic patterns in the cat.' *Archs Neurol., Chicago* **14**, 601–610

[28] Mahloudji, M. and Pikielny, R. T. (1967). 'Hereditary essential myoclonus.' *Brain* **90**, 669–674

[29] Metrakos, J. D. and Metrakos, K. (1960). 'Genetics of convulsive disorders I. Introduction, problems, methods and base lines. *Neurology* **10**, 228–240

[30] Metrakos, K. and Metrakos, J. D. (1961). 'Genetics of convulsive disorders II. Genetic and electroencephalographic studies in centrencephalic epilepsy.' *Neurology, Minneap.* **11**, 474–483

[31] Meyer, J. S., Gotoh, F. and Favale, E. (1966). 'Cerebral metabolism during epileptic seizures in man.' *Electroenceph. clin. Neurophysiol.* **21**, 10–22

[32] Milhorat, T. H. (1967). 'Experimental myoclonus of thalamic origin.' *Archs Neurol., Chicago* **17**, 365–378

[33] Noad, K. B. and Lance, J. W. (1960). 'Familial myoclonic epilepsy and its association with cerebellar disturbance.' *Brain* **83**, 618–630

[34] Penfield, W. P. and Jasper, H. H. (1954). *Epilepsy and the Functional Anatomy of the Human Brain.* Pp. 348–349. Boston; Little, Brown

[35] Pollen, D. A. (1964). 'Intracellular studies of cortical neurons during thalamic induced wave and spike.' *Electroenceph. clin. Neurophysiol.* **17**, 398–404

[36] Preswick, G., Reivich, M. and Hill, I. D. (1965). 'The E.E.G. effects of combined hyperventilation and hypoxia in normal subjects.' *Electroenceph. clin. Neurophysiol* **18**, 56–64

[37] Robb, P. (1965). 'Epilepsy. A review of basic and clinical research.' Monograph No. 1. National Institute of Neurological Diseases and Blindness. Bethesda, Maryland

[38] Rossi, G. F., Walter, R. D. and Crandall, P. H. (1968). 'Generalised spike and wave discharges and nonspecific thalamic nuclei.' *Archs Neurol., Chicago* **19**, 174–183

[39] Savage, D. C. L. (1967). 'Neurotoxic effects of piperazine.' *Br. med. J.* **1**, 840–841

[40] Symonds, C. P. (1953). 'Nocturnal myoclonus.' *J. Neurol. Neurosurg. Psychiat.* **16**, 166–171

[41] Symonds, C. P. (1959). 'Excitation and inhibition in epilepsy.' *Brain* **82**, 133–146

[42] Williams, D. (1965). 'The thalamus and epilepsy.' *Brain* **88**, 539–556

[43] Wohlfart, G. and Höök, O. (1951). 'A clinical analysis of myoclonus epilepsy (Unverricht-Lundborg), myoclonic cerebellar dyssynergy (Hunt) and hepato-lenticular degeneration (Wilson).' *Acta psychiat. neurol. scand.* **26**, 219–245

[44] Woodbury, D. M. (1958). 'Relation between the adrenal cortex and the central nervous system.' *Pharmac. Rev.* **10**, 275–357

11—The Relationship Between Brain and Mind

The understanding of mind is the central problem of man. Religious and political beliefs, scientific and cultural advances, the evaluation of life and of man's part in life depends upon concepts, products of the mind.

One's own mind is a subjective experience, a personal world which can be explored, within limits, by introspection. The mind of other men can be inferred from their speech, writing and actions, and the mind of animals from their actions alone. At what stage of the evolutionary scale is it justifiable to speak of mind, or indeed of consciousness? 'Refracted rearwards along the course of evolution, consciousness displays itself qualitatively as a spectrum of shifting hints whose lower terms are lost in the night.' (Teilhard de Chardin[36]).

A prerequisite for the phenomena of mind is consciousness, which may be described as a state in which there is the ability to be aware of sensation—that is, a state in which perception may take place. For purposes of discussion, components of mind may be considered as perception, memory, emotion, propositional thought and response (*Figure 11.1*). The nerve cells responsible for the act of perception are maintained in a state of readiness as a part of what is termed 'consciousness' by the ascending reticular activating system. When the system is in a state of awareness, the percept is registered, and by complex neuronal connexions is committed to memory. Percepts may then be correlated with pre-existing memory patterns and with the stored emotional content of those patterns. Effector or motor neurones then ensure that activity, whether it be speech or movement, can be initiated in a fashion appropriate to the information received. The end-products of the mind are apparent only in so far as they can be expressed in speech, writing or other action, which together constitute 'behaviour' in a broad sense.

'Personality' is the image of the subject evoked in the mind of the subject or other persons as the result of past and present patterns of behaviour. Personality can be altered by fatigue, hypoxia, hypoglycaemia, drugs, changes in the constitution of body fluids, or any local or general brain damage. The main purpose of the complex

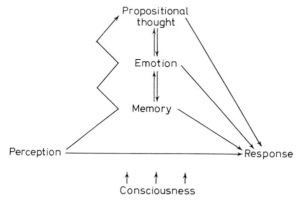

Figure 11.1. The elements of mind

homoeostatic mechanisms of the body is to keep the brain nourished by glucose and oxygen, and to provide the neurones with a suitable electrolyte solution in which to function, for it is in the brain that we have our being, and the other parts of the body are servants to it.

PERCEPTION

Man is made aware of his environment by the special senses of smell, vision and hearing, and can deduce his relationship to his surroundings by comparison with the memory of previous percepts. Additional information is obtained about objects close to him by the sensations of taste, touch, pressure, vibration, temperature discrimination and pain. Position and movement of the head in space is determined not only by vision, but by receptors in the vestibular system of the internal ear. The position of the body in relation to the head and to the ground is signalled by receptors in the joints and muscles, which also indicate the posture of the limbs. Thus man is provided with the mechanisms for sampling many of the physical properties of an external object, forming an holistic concept of it in his mind and placing it in a spatial and temporal relationship to himself and to other objects.

The act of perception is the transfer of information into its physicochemical equivalent in the appropriate part of the brain by propagation from sensory organs along nerve pathways to the sensory cortex[5]. The information may here be described as 'sense data' which are part of the perceptual world of the subject as distinct from the physical world of the object perceived[6]. Hallucinations of vision, hearing, smell and taste are not uncommon in disorders of the temporal lobe of the brain. At the same time as such a sensation is experienced, the electroencephalogram may show an electrical disturbance localized to the part of the brain whose abnormal activity is producing the sensation.

Two or even three stages of complexity may be recognized in such hallucinations affecting the special senses, particularly the senses of vision and hearing. The first is an unformed hallucination, such as flashes of coloured light or buzzing or humming noise. The second is a fragmentary sequence of events, organized but without context—the vision of a man moving or the brief snatch of a tune. The third is a development of the second, in which the visual or auditory hallucination tells a story in orderly sequence. The simplest form of hallucination derives from the primary receptive area for vision in the cortex of the occipital lobe of the brain, or that for hearing in the superior gyrus of the temporal lobe. More complex hallucinations probably originate in the temporal lobe, but the abnormal activity may spread through association fibres to other parts of the brain.

Penfield[26] has described the various psychical responses which may be obtained by electrical stimulation of the temporal lobes in the conscious patient. Many hallucinations have the same characteristics to the subject as normal sensations and thereby constitute percepts similar to those derived from external stimuli.

Continuous perception of stimuli is essential for neuronal events required in sequential thought. Removal of the afferent input to the cerebral cortex as in sensory deprivation experiments, leads to impairment of the normal thought processes. Subjects report an inability to concentrate, lack of clarity in thinking and difficulty in organizing their thoughts[44]. Under normal circumstances the brain is subjected to a continuous bombardment of afferent impulses, some of which may be relevant to a task of the moment, and others merely a distraction. At various levels in the nervous system, recurrent collaterals from afferent neurones synapse on neurones which inhibit adjacent afferent synapses, thus allowing a particular signal to take precedence in being perceived. This negative feedback, in electronic terms, diminishes the noise level and sharpens the discrimination[13]. This principle may in part explain the phenomenon of 'attention', whereby perception is selective.

MEMORY

The act of perception enables forms, figures, shapes, objects and ideas to be registered, or apprehended. These 'sense data' are stored, to be retrieved at will in temporal sequence.

Holofernes, in Shakespeare's *Love's Labours Lost*, says:

> This is a gift that I have, simple, simple; a foolish extravagant spirit, full of forms, figures, shapes, objects, ideas, apprehensions, motions, revolutions: these are begot in the ventricle of memory, nourished in the womb of pia mater, and delivered upon the mellowing of occasion. But the gift is good in those in whom it is acute, and I am thankful for it.

The precise mechanism of this simple gift so far eludes us.

The concept of Lashley[20] that lesions of equal area in different parts of the cortex have a comparable effect in retarding the learning process, has had to be revised, as excision of large areas of cortex in man may leave intellect and memory unimpaired, although these functions are vulnerable to smaller lesions in specific regions.

Entry portal for memory

It is probable that the registration of a memory takes place through the hippocampus and its connexions [2, 40]. Bilateral removal of the medial aspect of the temporal lobes produces an inability to record new experiences as well as some retrograde amnesia[33]. Removal of one temporal lobe does not alter the ability to memorize unless the other temporal lobe has been damaged previously, as in the two cases reported by Penfield and Milner[28]. On the other hand, stimulation of the temporal lobe, or epileptic seizures arising in the temporal lobe, can reproduce memory patterns.

Damage to the mammillary bodies and adjacent reticular formation is found in severe thiamine deficiency (Wernicke's encephalopathy), which is usually followed by a defect in recent memory and by confabulation (Korsakoff's syndrome). Confabulation is probably the result of a patient selecting random fragments of past events, for which the memory is intact, and using these to fill the gaps in recent memory without regard to time sequence.

If lesions of the hippocampus and mammillary bodies produce loss of recent memory, it is tempting to assume that the fornix which connects these structures may play its part in the establishment of memory. It is therefore important to note that the fornix may be divided surgically without loss of memory[40], unless there is associated damage to the region of the third ventricle[35].

The mammillothalamic tracts enter the anterior thalamic nuclei, which project to the frontal lobes and anterior cingulate gyri. Removal of both anterior cingulate gyri produces only an incomplete memory disturbance lasting about three days[41], and removal of, or damage to, one or both frontal lobes, does not produce any consistent change in memory[10]. It is possible that dorsomedial thalamic nuclei, which project to the frontal lobe, are part of the mechanism for retention of events for brief periods, as Schulman found that bilateral lesions grossly impaired the performance of monkeys in tests requiring a memory of up to 30 seconds[32].

It therefore appears that the hippocampi, mammillary bodies and adjacent reticular formation are essential for the registration of new memories, but the storage of old memories must involve extensive areas of the brain, since the memory of distant events is lost only when brain damage is diffuse, and even so, recent memory is always affected more than remote memory.

Long-term storage of memory

A memory trace, or 'engram', is usually implanted bilaterally in the cerebral cortex. Under experimental conditions, localization may be unilateral if the optic chiasm and corpus callosum have been divided ('split-brain animals'), and stimulation is restricted to the afferent connexions of one hemisphere[24] (*Figure 11.2*). Sperry[34] described how split-brain animals can be trained to respond to conflicting visual stimuli presented simultaneously, each hemisphere learning its own task independently. Removal of the cortex of one hemisphere, with sparing of 'islands' of cortex in specific areas, showed that the isolated visual cortex makes little contribution to visual learning and memory. On the other hand, the isolated sensorimotor cortex is capable of learning a variety of new somaesthetic discrimination patterns. Conditioned responses involving collaboration between cortical areas in both hemispheres may persist after extensive bisection of the brain extending down to the quadrigeminal plate, supporting the view of Gastaut[14] that brain-stem structures play an important part in conditioning. Russell and Ochs[30] blocked the function of one hemisphere for a period of days by the repeated topical application of a potassium chloride solution, and found that a memory trace was restricted permanently to the hemisphere active at the time of the learning process. If the function of each hemisphere were suppressed alternately after a conditioning process was completed, the memory was unimpaired; that is, an engram is laid down bilaterally under normal circumstances.

The nature of the neuronal change which marks the formation of a memory trace is not known. It may relay on physiological factors, a state of synaptic facilitation which is maintained by periodic reactivation of the neuronal circuit[12], or may require a

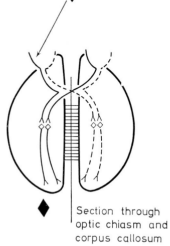

Figure 11.2. The split-brain preparation. Division of optic chiasm and corpus callosum ensures that a signal presented to the left eye is registered only in the left hemisphere (after Sperry[34])

Section through optic chiasm and corpus callosum

structural change in the nerve cell[31] and possibly its surrounding glial cells. Recently attention has become focused on ribonucleic acid (RNA) and desoxyribonucleic acid (DNA) as chemical mediators of memory. RNA is synthesized by the normal cell, its base sequence being specified by the genetic information in the DNA molecule.

Experimental work on planarians (flatworms) has produced evidence that memory is stored throughout the entire body of these worms, and furthermore that RNA may be involved in the storage process[21]. When a worm, which had been conditioned by an electric shock to respond to a light, was cut in half, the regenerated head and tail segments both retained the conditioned response. When the segments were allowed to regenerate in a solution containing ribonuclease, which destroys RNA, the tail segment forgot the response, but the head segment retained it. Most remarkable of all, if a conditioned worm were cut up and fed to an unconditioned worm, the worm would learn more rapidly than control worms.

This suggests that some chemical concerned in the memory process can be transmitted to another individual. These experiments have been followed by a number of negative attempts to reproduce them. More recently Ungar and Oceguera-Navarro[38] have claimed that mice injected with a peptide or small protein fraction of homogenized rat's brain habituated to a startle response much more rapidly when the donor animal had previously been habituated to the stimulus than when the donor animal was untrained.

The oral or intravenous administration of RNA to patients with disturbance of memory as a result of vascular disease or presenile or senile dementia has been stated to produce a significant improvement in performance in memory tests[8]. There is some evidence that the ribonuclease level is elevated in the blood of aged people with defects in memory, compared with normal controls.

The mechanism of memory storage may thus depend upon neurones being altered anatomically or chemically, or on being maintained in a state of activity so that the memory will not be lost. It has been suggested that the instructions for the synthesis of a memory-specific protein are contained in the genetic code-book like a digital computor program. When this is activated by an impinging electrical impulse, a set of genes is switched on to synthesize RNA which, in turn, directs the synthesis of cellular protein.

EMOTION

Emotion may be considered as having a sustained 'tonic' component and a relatively transient 'phasic' component, linked closely with autonomic activity. The tonic aspect of emotion sets the bias of reaction pattern, so that a person may be said to be of happy, amiable, irritable or gloomy disposition. The nature of this bias is not understood, although it can be altered readily by modern drugs, which may relieve (or produce) fear, anxiety and depression. The four classic humours may be found some day to have their counterparts in brain chemistry. Structural changes in the brain may also produce euphoria or depression; this implies that there is some anatomical correlation of emotional tonus.

The phasic aspect of emotion is a response to a perceived stimulus, and its nature depends upon memory of events associated with a similar percept; that is, it is a learned response. The emotional reaction of the maturing organism influences the selection of the appropriate motor response—grasping or avoiding, accepting or rejecting, caressing or fighting, advancing or retreating.

Stimulation and ablation experiments give some guide to the anatomical structures concerned with the expression of emotion in animals and man. Removal of the temporal lobe on both sides renders monkeys docile, with loss of fear and rage reactions[19]. A similar loss of affective reactions is seen in man after bitemporal lobectomy[37]. In the split-brain animal, these changes may be produced by a unilateral operation if the stimulus is presented solely to the operated hemisphere; that is, an animal may have a ferocious half-brain and a placid half-brain[34].

Decorticate cats show anger on slight provocation, the phenomenon known as 'sham rage'. If neocortex only is removed bilaterally, the animal is refractory to rage-provoking stimuli, a condition termed 'placidity' by Bard and Mountcastle[4]. The placid state is converted to one of ferocity by additional removal of transitional cortex of the midline or the pyriform lobes, amygdala and hippocampi. Bilateral ablations restricted to the amygdala and pyriform lobes produce a state of rage in which the animal retaliates by accurately attacking the source of irritation. Wheatley[39] had previously shown that destruction of the ventromedial hypothalamic nuclei would produce sham rage. Bard and Mountcastle concluded that an area extending from the hypothalamus to the amygdala was concerned with the inhibition of rage reactions in the cat.

The result of removing the amygdala is remarkably variable in different species, producing aggressive behaviour in cat and dog and a calming effect in monkey, opossum and rat[3], as well as in man.

Loss of fear reactions results from bilateral lesions of the dorsomedial thalamic nuclei, but not of the anterior thalamic nuclei, in the monkey[7]. The lack of affective reactions following damage to both frontal lobes in the human subject is probably a defect in the ability to project events in time, to 'visualize the consequences' of an act; that is, disturbance of emotion is a secondary phenomenon[10].

Epileptic seizures originating in the temporal lobes are frequently accompanied by a phasic emotional experience—fear, sadness, depression, pleasure or elation[42]. Such epileptic experiences are similar to those produced in man by electrical stimulation of the temporal lobe[27], but are cruder and more stereotyped than the wide range of emotions in the normal subject.

The emotional 'tonus' of an individual can be altered substantially by operations upon the amygdala and hypothalamic or thalamic nuclei, or upon the orbital surface of the frontal lobe. Although knowledge of the pathways serving emotion is so incomplete, the implication of temporal lobes and hypothalamus seems undeniable, with the frontal lobes playing some part as well.

RESPONSE

The simplest living organism will respond to external stimuli without the benefit of a nervous system. As the phylogenetic scale is ascended, specific cells are set aside for the reception of stimuli and the initiation of a response. The stretch reflex depends on two neurones only—a receptor and an effector neurone. Other reflexes employ intermediary neurones which may link together the cervical and lumbar outflow of the cord, so that the limb can be co-ordinated at a spinal level in movement such as walking. Others join brain-stem with spinal cord, so that the position of the head in relation to gravity can affect the posture of the limbs. Some simple reflexes such as placing reactions depend upon synaptic connexions in the cerebral cortex. Primitive 'startle responses', in which the subject moves suddenly when presented with a flash of light or loud noise, probably traverse the appropriate area of cerebral cortex and the reticular formation in the manner of a myoclonic jerk.

Conditioned reflexes may depend upon the thalamic reticular formation and thalamo-cortical connexions, rather than the cerebral cortex and cortico-cortical connexions as proposed by Pavlov[14]. Preservation of cortex is essential for initiating specific motor activity as part of a conditioned response, but an animal with all neocortex removed will still retain non-specific elements of a conditioned response—for example, changes in muscle tone, trembling and autonomic activity.

Further elaboration of the learning process must depend on correlation of a percept with a similar percept previously stored and memory of the temporal sequence of events which followed its acquisition. If there is a linkage retained between the stored percept and emotion, the memory gives rise to a sense of pleasure or displeasure, thus giving a personal sign to the stored percept. The reaction of the organism is then altered accordingly, so that a reaction pattern of 'acceptance' or 'rejection' can be set in motion. The frontal lobes appear to be necessary for comprehension of the total significance of a situation and appreciation of the possible consequences of an act, so that the response may be appropriate to the situation, even though memory and emotion may remain intact after damage to the frontal lobes[10].

The simplest patterns of acceptance or rejection can be seen in infants before they become conditioned responses, and they can be seen in isolated form in an adult when they are released by focal brain damage from their normal state of inhibition. These responses are known as the 'grasp reflex' and the 'avoiding reaction'. If the medial aspect of the frontal lobes have been destroyed, the human patient will grasp firmly any object drawn down the palm from wrist to fingers. Indeed, the patient may grope towards any object presented to him and then grasp it.

The contrary is seen if the lateral aspect of the parietal lobe is injured, when a light stimulus applied to the hand will lead to extension of the fingers and wrist, and withdrawal of the hand. These conflicting reactions of acceptance and rejection are normally mediated through the basal ganglia and held in balance by cortical function. They are released by damage to the cortex or basal ganglia[11].

We have considered the conditioned response and the elaboration of this in which the emotional content of stored percepts leads to expression in one of two divergent directions as acceptance or rejection. It is fairly easy to proceed from this to a reasoned response, based on judgment, which in turn must involve the correlation of a vast number of memory traces. This process is easier to understand when we see the way in which a computer can correlate the information stored on a number of magnetic tapes. The response is obviously much more complex than the basic patterns of acceptance and rejection outlined above, although complex behaviour comprises combinations of motor activity in which simple stereotyped responses may be detected. Furthermore, complex motor performance may be altered while it is in progress by feedback of information to the nervous system to adjust the nature of the activity to a changing situation. Patients with dorsolateral frontal lobe damage are unable to shift rapidly from one principle to another, and will persist with an outmoded response, although recognizing that their actions are inappropriate[22].

PROPOSITIONAL THOUGHT

A higher form of intellectual endeavour, logical or propositional thought, proceeds from a given premise to a conclusion. Here memory may provide the premise which then acts as an internal stimulus, taking the place of a perceived stimulus, to initiate a chain of events. Propositional thought is the basis of what we term intelligence, a general impression of intellectual ability comprising an aggregation of special skills, each of which may be developed to a different degree in the one person. Damage to certain parts of the brain is associated with specific forms of intellectual disability, which are more frequent with left hemisphere lesions than right, and with posterior lesions than anterior. These syndromes are considered in detail by Piercy[29], who makes it clear that different parts of the brain are not equipotential for intelligence, and throws doubt on the concept of 'general intelligence' over and above the correlation of specific abilities.

The finest flowering of propositional thought, and the hardest to conceive in mechanistic terms, is original or creative thought. How is it possible for a symphony to be born of a computer? Suppose that a man of musically talented stock, who has the genetic gift of special receptors and neuronal circuits appropriate for the perception and storage of musical tunes, determines to compose an original work. He has in his memory countless tunes written by others, as well as sounds heard in nature and mathematical concepts which he has learned or developed in the past. It does not seem impossible that the simultaneous activation of all the relevant neuronal connexions would lead to the selection of a sequence of notes, harmonies and rhythms which then form a completely new tune, regarded as 'original' by all who subsequently hear it. Jefferson[18] expressed the same thought attractively as follows.

> If our minds were capable of the pure inventions which our pride tells us is the case, why, sir or madam, do you not add to the sum of human knowledge by some flash of intuitive reasoning far outside your usual orbit, make some mathematical postulation, provide some explanation in atomic physics, some statement on molecular structure in physical chemistry, some new discovery in astrophysics or in biology, and some superb musical composition or work of art such as would not only win the world's approval, not only gratify but certainly astonish your friends? You will have to confess that you yourself would be greatly surprised by such a creation. The reason is clear—that discovery is only to be made by those who have put into their heads the material necessary for discovery or have assiduously practised skills.

Although we are far from understanding the mechanism of creative thought, we know enough to consider it in materialistic terms, as a product of neuronal function. It does not seem possible to regard it otherwise when one observes the gradual restriction of thought processes occurring in a brilliant man who has been afflicted with some form of progressive cerebral disease. As the brain is altered and its nerve-cells wither, the patient's expression in speech, writing and other action deteriorates. His relatives and friends say that his behaviour and personality have changed. All the qualities which stamped the man as an individual spirit become blurred and indefinite. As Cohen[9] puts it:

> Experience soon teaches us that there is no accepted attribute of mind such as purpose, reasoning, thought, memories, feeling, willing, which cannot be disturbed by brain disease, that there are no abnormalities of mind whose special features allow associated brain disease to be excluded. There is, that is to say, no way of excluding the presence of cerebral pathology from the

most exact appraisal of mental symptoms alone, be they defects of memory or concentration as feeling, hallucinations, illusions or delusions, or a host of other manifestations of disease which we label 'mental'.

DEMENTIA

When faced with the problem of apparent intellectual deterioration, one must determine first whether one is dealing with a psychiatric disturbance such as a depressive state, a transient impairment of mental acuity such as a toxi-confusional state, a focal cerebral lesion, multi-focal cerebral lesions, or a global cortical atrophy. The distinction between these groups becomes blurred since prolonged toxic states may lead to irreversible brain damage, and one or more focal cerebral lesions may destroy large areas of cortex so that their localized nature is obscured and all forms of mental ability seem to be equally afflicted.

A suitable pragmatic approach is to consider first the causes of organic mental change which are potentially remediable.

(1) Intoxications: alcohol, bromides, barbiturates and various anticonvulsant drugs, and agents used in the treatment of Parkinson's disease. Infections, for example, of the urinary tract, are liable to cause mental confusion in the elderly or disabled patient.

(2) Metabolic abnormalities:
Hypoglycaemia. Hypocalcaemia or hypercalcaemia. Respiratory, renal and hepatic failure. Vitamin B_{12} deficiency, which may be responsible for mental changes before any alteration in the peripheral blood picture, or other signs of neurological disturbance such as peripheral neuropathy or subacute combined degeneration. Nicotinic acid deficiency—pellagra. Thiamine deficiency—Wernicke's encephalopathy, seen commonly in alcoholic patients. Porphyria.

(3) Endocrine abnormalities: Myxoedema, thyrotoxicosis, Addison's disease, Cushing's syndrome. A phaeochromocytoma producing more adrenaline than noradrenaline may stimulate an anxiety state.

(4) Chronic infections such as neurosyphilis.

(5) Space-occupying lesions: Tumours, particularly of frontal and temporal lobes, for example, olfactory groove meningioma. Subdural haematoma may rarely produce confusion before drowsiness and headache.

(6) Non-communicating hydrocephalus.

(7) Communicating hydrocephalus. Adams and his colleagues[1] have recently pointed out that absorption of cerebrospinal fluid may become defective following head injury or subarachnoid haemorrhage, or spontaneously in middle-aged or elderly persons.

It has long been known that adhesive arachnoiditis could prevent the passage of c.s.f. over the convexity of the cerebral hemispheres in conditions such as tuberculous meningitis. Now that it is recognized that the subarachnoid space may become obliterated without any obvious causative illness, it is worthwhile performing pneumoencephalography on any patient with mental impariment. If the lateral ventricles are dilated but air fails to enter the subarachnoid space after repeated attempts, there is presumptive evidence of communicating hydrocephalus and a shunt between the lateral ventricles and atrium via the jugular vein may produce worthwhile improvement

Most cerebral disease in its advanced stages will cause dementia, and there are some specific patterns of neuronal degeneration, such as the presenile dementias, which are irremediable in the present state of knowledge.

FOCAL CEREBRAL SYMPTOMS

The cerebral cortex is responsible for the content of consciousness and for the many components of mental ability, which in the aggregate we call 'intellect'. It is often possible to find a specific loss of certain mental skills in a patient who has been thought to be dementing, and thus to localize a lesion to one particular area of cerebral cortex.

Many of the skills, such as speech, writing and calculation, are usually restricted to one cerebral hemisphere, thus leading to the concept of dominance of one hemisphere, which in turn is linked with handedness. Lateralization of speech functions has been studied in large numbers of patients with unilateral brain disease, injury or focal epilepsy, with the general conclusion that the great majority of right-handed subjects are left-brained for speech, as are more than half of the left-handed subjects. Speech function in the remaining left-handers is controlled by the right half of the brain or distributed between the hemispheres. In recent years, the technique of injecting amylobarbitone into the internal carotid artery has been used to determine cerebral dominance. By this method, Milner, Branch and Rasmussen[23] showed that of 44 left-handed subjects without any evidence of left hemisphere damage, speech was represented on the left in 28 (64 per cent), bilaterally in 7 (16 per cent) and on the right in 9 (20 per cent). There was evidence of previous left hemisphere damage in another 27 subjects, in whom the distribution was reversed, 6 (22 per cent) having speech function in the left hemisphere, 3 (11 per cent) bilaterally, and 18 (67 per cent) on the right side.

Presumably the two groups correspond broadly to genetic and acquired left-handedness.

The posterior part of the temporal lobe, behind Heschl's gyrus, is larger on the left in 65 per cent of brains, and larger on the right in only 11 per cent[16]. The area at the junction of the parietal and temporal lobes of the brain, incorporating the supramarginal and angular gyri, is the 'black box' of the dominant hemisphere, the association area of association areas (*Figure 11.3*). It is the centre for the integration of sensory information, particularly from the special senses of hearing and vision, and for the formulation of an

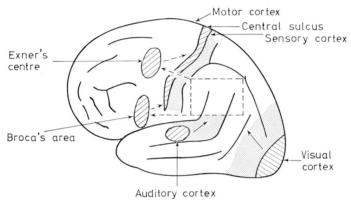

Figure 11.3. Schema of the mechanism for speech and writing in the dominant hemisphere. The area at the junction of the parietal lobe and posterior temporal lobes, which is marked as a square by an interrupted line, is situated between the auditory, visual and sensory association areas and receives projections from them. The internal formulation of speech and writing takes place within this area which is connected with a motor association area lying anterior to the motor strip. Subsidiary centres for speech and writing in the motor association area then transmit the appropriate neural pattern to face and hand areas of the motor cortex respectively

appropriate response through speech, writing or other actions. The 'black box' is strategically situated between the association areas for hearing, vision and common sensation, and is connected with the frontal lobes for translation of a planned response into action. There is a subsidiary speech area (Broca's area) in the frontal lobe anterior to that part of the motor cortex which is concerned with movements of the face and tongue. Broca's area may be considered as a final integrating centre for speech mechanisms before the motor cortex and corticobulbar fibres transmit the appropriate pattern to the cranial nerves responsible for speech. It is probable that there is an integrating centre for writing, comparable with Broca's area for speech, situated anterior to the hand area of the motor cortex and known as Exner's writing centre[25]. It is attractive to postulate that similar integrating centres for other forms of skilled movement also lie anterior to the motor cortex, since it is known that frontal lobe lesions, as well as parietal lobe lesions, may lead to difficulty in performing movements, even those which are semi-automatic such as walking, in the absence of any impairment of motor pathways. The concept is thus developed of a parieto-temporal integrating centre which abstracts information from the sensory association areas, and projects forward to what might be termed a motor association area where the neural patterns for speech, writing and skilled movement are programmed for transmission down corticobulbar and corticospinal tracts. Breakdown in the mechanism for speech (dysphasia, aphasia), writing (dysgraphia, agraphia) or skilled movement (dyspraxia, apraxia) may be attributed to disconnexion of association areas[15]. Apraxia may result from lesions of association areas lying anterior to the motor cortex, from lesions in the region of the supramarginal gyrus, or to damage to association fibres connecting these areas, including the corpus callosum.

On the receptive side, damage to the sensory association areas or their connexions with the speech area of the dominant hemisphere causes inadequacy in reading (dyslexia, alexia), in recognition of the spoken word (auditory agnosia or sensory aphasia) and in identification of common sensations (agnosia) without any disorder in the primary sensory system. Geschwind regards most 'agnosias' as modality-specific naming defects resulting from isolation of the primary sensory cortex from the speech area, often associated with a confabulatory response[15].

A lesion in the region of the supramarginal and angular gyri will cause defects in comprehension as well as defects in expression, that is, a mixed sensory and motor aphasia in the case of speech mechanisms, and the whole internal organisation of speech may be destroyed. In contrast, a lesion of Broca's area will affect word selection and expression but recognition of speech and 'internal speech' remains intact. A lesion of the black box area may cause difficulty in calculations (acalculia) and right-left disorientation as well as dysgraphia and language disorders.

Lesions of the non-dominant parietal lobe may produce an apraxia for constructional tasks or for dressing, and the patient may neglect the left half of space and the left side of his own body, even denying that his left arm and leg belong to him. This type of disturbance is rarely seen in lesions of the dominant hemisphere, possibly because the connexions from sensory association areas to central integrating centre are shorter and less complex than those from the non-dominant hemisphere which have to cross in the corpus callosum[15].

The specialized functions which have just been discussed may be impaired temporarily by focal epileptic discharge, migrainous vasospasm, or insufficiency of the internal carotid artery. They may be permanently damaged by trauma, encephalitis, cortical infarction or compression by an expanding lesion. It is important that such symptoms be recognized as an indication of localized brain damage, and that the cause be sought, since many are remediable.

The posterior cerebral arteries, which receive most of their blood supply from the basilar artery, supply the medial aspects of both temporal lobes and occipital cortex. For this reason it is not uncommon for loss of memory to be a symptom of basilar artery insufficiency, since both hippocampal regions are rendered ischaemic or infarcted at the time. Such episodes are usually accompanied by blurring of vision, uniformed visual hallucinations, or cortical blindness, as well as symptoms of brain-stem dysfunction, such as vertigo, dysarthria, ataxia, bilateral paraesthesiae or weakness.

THE INFLUENCE OF THE MIND ON THE BODY

The brain's dominion extends to the extremities of the body, through the peripheral and autonomic nervous system, and the secretions of those endocrine glands which are under neural control. The neural centres for simple vegetative functions are found within the brain-stem and hypothalamus. Superimposed on these is the limbic system, a phylogenetically old ring of cortex which loops around the corpus callosum and third ventricle, including the cingulate gyrus, hippocampus and amygdaloid nucleus. In control of the limbic cortex is the neocortex, which makes up the bulk of the brain in man. Of particular significance in emotional reactions are the orbital surface of the frontal lobe and the temporal lobe, as described earlier.

Failure of adaptation to stress renders man liable to a variety of diseases which are caused, or at least aggravated, by mental processes. Overaction of neck, jaw, facial and scalp muscles is largely responsible for tension headache and also plays a part in increasing the frequency of migraine attacks. Periodic swelling of the nasal mucosa, vasomotor rhinitis, may be a response to anxiety as well as to irritant fumes or allergies[43]. In a similar manner, the bronchi may constrict under conditions of stress or excitement and the bronchial mucosa then excretes excessive mucus, a state characteristic of asthma. A more direct association with stress is seen in the overbreathing of acute anxiety reactions. Overbreathing may be prolonged to such an extent that tetany supervenes, because the alkalosis of hypocapnia induces a deficiency of ionised calcium in the blood. The subject experiences distal and facial paraesthesiae and the muscles of upper and lower limbs may pass into a state of tetanic contraction. The posture of the limbs, with flexion at metacarpo-phalangeal joints and extension of the interphalangeal joints (*Figure 11.4*) and rigid plantar flexion and inversion of the feet, is presumably determined by anatomical factors, the stronger muscles overcoming the weaker,

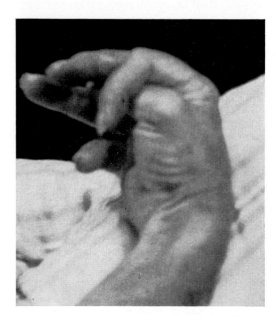

Figure 11.4. Tetanic spasm of the hand occurring in hypocalcaemia, or when the level of ionized calcium is diminished by overbreathing in an acute anxiety reaction

since all peripheral nerves would be equally hyperactive in the hypocalcaemic state. The posture is the same as that seen in the tonic phase of seizures and in the dystonia which results from progressive extrapyramidal disease, or as a late result of a hemiplegia. It is the end-point of a nonselective increase in motor activity whether the cause be central or peripheral. Overbreathing also causes a feeling of faintness, and mild sustained overbreathing or 'sighing' respiration is a common mechanism of psychogenic vertigo, or 'light-headedness'.

The gastrointestinal tract is profoundly influenced by emotion. The mouth dries up in situations of stress, in a final viva voce examination, or at the beginning of an important speech. On the other hand, salivary excretion may be increased in states of anxiety or depression ('ptyalism'). The stomach has two distinct reaction

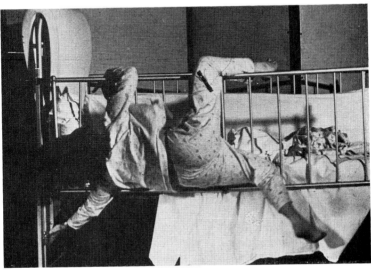

Figure 11.5. The climax of an hysterical fit. After thrashing about in bed, the patient habitually hurled herself over the bed rails and continued the attack with swimming movements on the floor

patterns, the first with hyperaemia and engorgement of the mucosa, increased secretion of HCl and motor activity, and the second with pallor of the mucosa, and depressed secretion and motility[43]. The former state, which may be induced by resentment or hostility, is commonly associated with duodenal ulcer. The latter state may be an accompaniment of depression or the 'anorexia nervosa' of hysteria. Functional diarrhoea may be a symptom of excitement, anxiety or inadequate adjustment to life's problems. Conversely, constipation may occur in hysterical or depressive states.

Anxiety may play a part in cardiac extrasystoles, hypertension and coronary heart disease. It is the commonest cause of impotence. It may provoke frequency of micturition or retention of urine. Anxiety may underlie the complaints of backache, dysmenorrhoea, obesity or eczema.

233

Hysterical states may produce symptoms and signs which mimic those of neurological disease, ranging through polyuria from compulsive water-drinking, blindness, deafness, amnesic fugues, anaesthesia and paralysis to grotesque movement disorders and hysterical fits (*Figure 11.5*). It is necessary to make a positive diagnosis of hysteria by considering the patient's personality, life situation, and psychological escape mechanisms, rather than making a diagnosis solely by exclusion of organic disease. Inconsistencies in the physical examination often assist the diagnosis. For example, a patient with hysterical 'deafness' is often under the impression that the ear being blocked by the examiner's finger is the ear being tested, and thus hears in the 'deaf' ear and appears to be deaf in the normal ear.

The unity of cerebral and bodily function makes it essential to consider each patient as an individual living in his own world, with his distinctive reactions to the joys and hardships of his own life. The good neurologist does not regard his patient as a nervous system in aspic.

GENERAL CONCLUSIONS

Knowledge of the physical basis of mental function is incomplete, but the outline can be seen. The unity of brain and mind is apparent to any who observe the effect of brain damage, as a single focal lesion, as a sequence of events in different areas of the cerebral cortex or as the progression of a diffuse atrophic change. The developing child shows day by day evidence of increasing complexity of intellectual function. The brain-stricken adult shows day by day a diminution of this power. As the brain changes in structure, all the qualities which we recognize collectively as personality are changed with it. It is harder for man to accept the temporal limitations inherent in a materialistic view of intellect and spirit, than it is to accept the vulnerability of other bodily functions. This is doubtless the reason for the development and persistence of the religious or supernatural concept of a soul, whose entity is undisturbed by death of the brain and its bodily framework. Hebb stated: 'In the twilight zone between neurology and philosophy, for example, there is a group of writers who seem emotionally committed to a defence of the soul as against any mechanistic theory of man'[17]. He points out that 'there is no neuropsychological theory at present that does not have grave defects, and thus no danger that such theory will "disprove" the theory of an immaterial mind or soul, for a long time to come at least. One's beliefs therefore need not prejudice one's choice of working method'.

234

Whatever one's views, one can find satisfaction in the ability of man to store information outside his brain. The library acts as a universal memory for mankind. Moreover, the expression of neuronal activity as a concept which may be transferred to the minds of others can result in events which are propagated far beyond the lifetime of the brain which generated the concept. Finally, the transmission of neuronal pattern through gene chemistry from generation to generation ensures that the individual becomes one with the future development of man.

SUMMARY

Mind is the product of the conscious brain and has been considered in a number of its aspects which interact one with the other. The entry portal for memory is the hippocampal region, and the registration of memory is impaired when this area is damaged bilaterally, for example, in basilar artery insufficiency. Long-term memory is laid down diffusely and bilaterally under normal circumstances but may be restricted to one hemisphere when the optic chiasm and corpus callosum are divided (split-brain preparation) and perception is limited to that hemisphere. Emotional reactions may be altered by selective cerebral ablation, an extreme example being seen in a split-brain animal, which can be prepared with a ferocious half-brain and a placid half-brain.

The emotional association of a perceived event, which derives from memory of similar events, will not only affect the storage of that particular event in memory, but may also affect the act of perception itself. Memory storage may depend upon synthesis of RNA, its base sequence being specified by the genetic information in the DNA molecule. The extent and quality of memory traces laid down, and the degree of association between them, provide the substance for propositional thought. Response is biassed towards acceptance or rejection by the prevailing emotional tone of the subject, which may be influenced by fatigue, hypoxia, hypoglycaemia, drugs, vitamin deficiency, the constitution of body fluids, the endocrine glands, or by local or general brain damage.

In a patient whose intellect has deteriorated one must determine whether the defect involves all modalities, for example, a toxi-confusional state or dementia, or whether the symptoms are those of a focal cortical lesion. The integration of sensory information and certain tools of intellect, among them speech, writing and skilled movement, are mediated by a relatively small area of the dominant hemisphere. A precise clinical assessment is required to dissect focal from general changes, and to diagnose the remediable causes of organic mental change. The mind influences bodily reactions and many disorders of the respiratory, gastrointestinal and other systems are caused or aggravated by mental processes. The relation of brain to mind and mind to body remains one of the most fascinating and one of the most important problems in medicine.

REFERENCES

[1] Adams, R. D., Fisher, C. M., Hakim, S., Ojemann, R. G. and Sweet, W. H. (1965). 'Symptomatic occult hydrocephalus with "normal" cerebrospinal fluid pressure.' *New Engl. J. Med.* **273**, 117–126

[2] Barbizet, J. (1963). 'Defect of memorizing of hippocampal-mammillary origin: A review.' *J. Neurol. Neurosurg. Psychiat.* **26**, 127–135

[3] Bard, P. (1958). In Ciba Foundation Symposium, *Neurological Basis of Behaviour*, pp. 234–235. London; Churchill

[4] Bard, P. and Mountcastle, V. B. (1948). 'Some forebrain mechanisms involved in expression of rage with special reference to suppression of angry behaviour.' *Res. Publs. Ass. nerv. ment. Dis.* **27**, 362–404

[5] Brain, W. R. (1951). *Mind, Perception and Science.* Oxford; Blackwell

[6] Brain, W. R. (1959). *The Nature of Experience.* London; Oxford University Press

[7] Brierley, J. B. and Beck, E. (1958). 'The effects upon behaviour of lesions in the dorsomedial and anterior thalamic nuclei of cat and monkey.' In Ciba Foundation Symposium, *Neurological Basis of Behaviour*, pp. 90–104. London; Churchill

[8] Cameron, D. E. (1963). 'The process of remembering.' *Br. J. Psychiat.* **109**, 325–340

[9] Cohen, J. (1952). 'The status of brain in the concept of mind.' *Philosophy* **27**, 195–210

[10] Denny-Brown, D. (1951). 'The frontal lobes and their functions.' In *Modern Trends in Neurology*, pp. 13–89. Ed. by A. Feiling. London; Butterworths

[11] Denny-Brown, D. (1962). *The Basal Ganglia and their Relation to Disorders of Movement.* London; Oxford University Press

[12] Eccles, J. C. (1953). *The Neurophysiological Basis of Mind*, p. 227. Oxford; Clarendon

[13] Eccles, J. C. (1964). 'The controls of sensory communication to the brain.' *Australas. Ann. Med.* **13**, 102–113

[14] Gastaut, H. (1958). 'Some aspects of the neurophysiological basis of conditioned reflexes and behaviour.' In Ciba Foundation Symposium *Neurological Basis of Behaviour*, pp. 255–276. London; Churchill

[15] Geschwind, N. (1965). 'Disconnexion syndromes in animals and man.' *Brain* **88**, 237–294, 585–644

[16] Geschwind, N. and Levitsky, W. (1968). 'Human brain: left-right asymmetries in temporal speech region.' *Science, N.Y.* **161**, 186–187

[17] Hebb, D. O. (1958). 'Intelligence, brain function and the theory of mind.' *Brain* **82**, 260–275

[18] Jefferson, G. (1955). 'Meditations on the sources of knowledge.' *Lancet* **2**, 935–937

[19] Klüver, H. and Bucy, P. C. (1937). 'Psychic blindness and other symptoms following bilateral temporal lobectomy in Rhesus monkeys.' *Am. J. Physiol.* **119**, 352–353

[20] Lashley, K. S. (1937). 'Functional determinates of cerebral localization.' *Archs Neurol. Psychiat., Chicago* **38**, 371–387

[21] McConnell, J. V. (1962). 'Memory transfer through cannibalism in planarians.' *J. Neuropsychiat.* **3**, Suppl. 1, S42–48

[22] Milner, B. (1963). 'Effects of different brain lesions on card sorting.' *Archs Neurol., Chicago* **9**, 90–100

[23] Milner, B., Branch, C. and Rasmussen, T. (1964). 'Observations on cerebral dominance.' In *Disorders of Language*. Ciba Foundation Symposium Ed. by A. V. S. de Reuck and M. O'Connor. London; Churchill

[24] Myers, R. E. (1956). 'Function of corpus callosum in interocular transfer.' *Brain* **79**, 358–363

[25] Nielsen, J. M. (1946). *Agnosia, Apraxia, Aphasia. Their Value in Cerebral Localization*. New York; Hoeber

[26] Penfield, W. (1958). 'The role of the temporal cortex in recall of past experience and interpretation of the present.' In Ciba Foundation Symposium *Neurological Basis of Behaviour*, pp. 149–174. London; Churchill

[27] Penfield, W. and Jasper, H. (1954). *Epilepsy and the Functional Anatomy of the Human Brain*. Boston; Little, Brown

[28] Penfield, W. and Milner, B. (1958). 'Memory deficit produced by bilateral lesions in the hippocampal zone.' *Archs Neurol. Psychiat. Chicago* **79**, 475–497

[29] Piercy, M. (1964). 'The effects of cerebral lesions on intellectual function: A review of current research trends.' *Br. J. Psychiat.* **110**, 310–352

[30] Russell, I. S. and Ochs, S. (1963). 'Localization of a memory trace in one cortical hemisphere and transfer to the other hemisphere.' *Brain* **86**, 37–54

[31] Russell, W. R. (1959). *Brain. Memory. Learning*, p. 79. London; Oxford University Press

[32] Schulman, S. (1964). 'Impaired delayed response from thalamic lesions.' *Archs Neurol., Chicago* **11**, 477–499

[33] Scoville, W. B. and Milner, B. (1957). 'Loss of recent memory after bilateral hippocampal lesions.' *J. Neurol. Neurosurg. Psychiat.* **20**, 11–21

[34] Sperry, R. W. (1961). 'Cerebral organization and behaviour.' *Science, N.Y.* **133**, 1749–1757

[35] Sweet, W. H. Talland, G. A. and Ervin, F. R. (1959). 'Loss of recent memory following section of fornix.' *Trans. Am. neurol. Ass.* **84**, 76–82

[36] Teilhard de Chardin, P. (1959). *The Phenomenon of Man*, p. 59. Translated by B. Wall. London; Collins

[37] Terzian, H. and Dalle Ore, G. (1955). 'Syndrome of Klüver and Bucy reproduced in man by bilateral removal of the temporal lobes.' *Neurology, Minneap.* **5**, 373–380

[38] Ungar, G. and Oceguera-Navarro, C. (1965). 'Transfer of habitation by material extracted from the brain.' *Nature, Lond.* **207**, 301–302

[39] Wheatley, M. D. (1944). 'The hypothalamus and affective behaviour in cats. A study of the effects of experimental lesions with anatomic correlations.' *Archs Neurol. Psychiat., Chicago* **52**, 296–316

[40] Whitty, C. W. M. (1962). 'The neurological basis of memory.' In *Modern Trends in Neurology*—3, pp. 314–335. London; Butterworths

[41] Whitty, C. W. M. and Lewin, W. (1960). 'A Korsakoff syndrome in the post-cingulectomy confusional state.' *Brain* **83**, 648–653

[42] Williams, D. (1956). 'The structure of emotions reflected in epileptic experiences.' *Brain* **79**, 29–67

[43] Wolff, H. G. (1968). *Stress and Disease*. Ed. by S. Wolf and H. Goodell. Springfield; Thomas

[44] Zubek, J. P. (1964). 'Effects of prolonged sensory and perceptual deprivation.' *Br. med. Bull.* **20**, 38–42

INDEX

Acceptance and rejection, 224
Acetylcholine, neuromuscular
    transmission and, 36
    synaptic transmission and, 193
Acoustic neuroma, 169
Alcohol, cerebellar disease, causing,
    151, 158
Amygdala, emotions, effect on, 223
Anoxia, athetosis, causing, 133
    basal ganglia, effect on, 124
    (*see also* Hypoxia)
Aorta, thrombosis of, 31, 32
Archicerebellar syndrome, 151
Archicerebellum, 145
Arm,
    dermatomes and sclerotomes, 9
    weakness of, 30
Arnold-Chiari malformation, 156
Asthenia, 28
Ataxia,
    cerebellar disease, in, 151, 155
    vestibular damage, in, 165
Athetosis, 132
Auditory artery thrombosis, 168

Babinski response, 108
Backache, 22
Basal ganglia, 120–143
    anoxia, effect of, 124
    athetosis, role in, 133
    disease of,
        dystonia in, 136

Basal ganglia—*cont.*
    Parkinson's disease, role in, 127
    righting reflex, and, 123
    siezures in, 199
Basilar artery insufficiency, 187, 231
Békésy audiometry, 176
Bladder, pain in, 15
Bowel pain, 14
Brachial plexus, injury to, 33, 34
Brachial radiculitis, 15
Bradykinin, 24
Brain,
    damage, memory loss, causing,
        220
    haematoma, 30, 186
    infections, consciousness, loss of,
        causing, 186
    intelligence and, 225
    relationship to mind, 216
    senile disease, 131
    tumours,
        convulsions in, 200
        dementia, causing, 227
        transient paresis, causing, 44
Brain-stem,
    compression, 186
    lesions, vertigo, causing, 169
Broca's area, 229
Brown-Séquard syndrome, 20, 30

Endocrine disorders,
dementias, causing, 227
muscular weakness in, 41, 46
Endorgans,
muscle spindle fibres, in, 52
sensation and, 3
Endplate potential, 36
Epilepsy,
consciousness, loss of, 188
extrapyramidal, 138
familial myoclonic, 159
hereditary tendency, 194
mechanism of, 193
myoclonus in, 204, 206
neuronal activity, 193, 198
petit mal, 45, 188
seizures,
emotion and, 223
factors causing, 196
focal, 199
grand mal (major), 199
mechanism, 199
petit mal, 205
prevention, 198
toxic, 199
synaptic transmission in, 193, 198
temporal lobe, vertigo, causing,
171
emotions in, 201, 223
Extensor plantar response, 108
Extrapyramidal motor system, 120
disorders,
dystonia and, 138
rigidity in, 110
epileptic fits, in, 203
hemiballismus and, 129
Extrapyramidal tracts,
effects on stretch reflex, 78
Eyes,
vertigo, as cause of, 171
vestibular connexions, 166

Face,
pain in, 6
Familial cerebellar atrophy, 159
Fasciculation, 32
Flexor reflex, 11
control of, 90

Flexor reflex—cont.
initiation, 108
Fore brain
damage to, 50
Formication, 2
Frontal lobe, 226

Gait, 68
cerebellar disease, in, 151, 155
pyramidal tract section, effect of,
82
vestibular damage, in, 165
Gall bladder disease, 14
Gamma efferent system, 52
Gastro-intestinal pain, 14
Globus pallidus, 122, 123
Golgi tendon organs, 54
Guillain–Barré syndrome, 34, 46

Haematomyelia, 32
Hamstring jerk, 59, 60
Hand,
muscle wasting, 33, 36
Hartnup disease, 156
Head,
injury, cerebellar disease, causing,
156
movements,
control of, 122
perception of, 165
position in space, 217
effects of, 73
perception of, 163
Headache,
causes, 12
management of, 22
tension, 17, 22, 24
Hearing tests, 176
Heart,
pain in, 13, 22
sensory fibres from, 10
Hemiballismus, 128
Hemiparesis, transient, 44
Hemiplegia, 30
Herpes zoster, 16
Hippocampus memory, and, 219
Hoffmann's sign, 63
Hydrocephalus, 227